FAST

THIS WAY

FAST
THIS WAY

BURN FAT, HEAL INFLAMMATION, AND EAT LIKE THE
HIGH-PERFORMING HUMAN YOU WERE MEANT TO BE

DAVE ASPREY

HARPER WAVE
An Imprint of HarperCollins*Publishers*

FIRST EDITION

Library of Congress Cataloging-in-Publication Data

Names: Asprey, Dave, author.
Title: Fast this way : how to lose weight, get smarter, and live your longest, healthiest life with the bulletproof guide to fasting / Dave Asprey.
Description: First edition. | New York City: Harper Wave, 2021. | Includes bibliographical references and index.
Identifiers: LCCN 2020039140 (print) | LCCN 2020039141 (ebook) | ISBN 9780062882868 (hardcover) | ISBN 9780062882882 (ebook)
Subjects: LCSH: Intermittent fasting. | Weight loss. | Longevity.
Classification: LCC RM222.2 .A8367 2021 (print) | LCC RM222.2 (ebook) | DDC 613.2/5--dc23
LC record available at https://lccn.loc.gov/2020039140
LC ebook record available at https://lccn.loc.gov/2020039141

21 22 23 24 25 LSC   10 9 8 7 6 5 4 3 2 1

To my lovely wife, Dr. Lana, who is most definitely not

spending her time cooking breakfast anymore

CONTENTS

FAST

THIS WAY

PROLOGUE: FASTING TO FIND YOUR BEST SELF

The shaman's instructions were quite specific: bring only a sleeping bag, a flashlight, water, and a knife for the vision quest. The first three items were critical for my survival. The last one was mostly for my peace of mind, apparently, because the biggest danger near my cave was coyotes, and coyotes don't usually attack people. But on this kind of journey, there's no simple boundary between physical and psychological well-being. Is there ever, really?

I had set off on my first vision quest in search of better health, greater self-awareness, and, above all, in the hope of achieving a deeper sense of peace. To an outside observer, I looked like a man who had found his success. It was in 2008, four years after my travels to Tibet and Mount Kailash, where I first learned about the mind-bending qualities of yak butter tea. There was a time when I wore size 46 pants and weighed more than 300 pounds, but that was behind me. After failing at every diet there was, I had invented a new one and had lost most of the weight I wanted to lose. I'd pushed myself into good physical condition. I was busily learning about ways to hack the body, seeking out new methods to radically enhance my energy, my abilities, and my longevity. I had already begun developing the concept for Bulletproof Coffee, the company I would start a couple years later.

Outside appearances are not what truly define us, however. On the inside, I was dealing with unsatisfied cravings in many different forms. I felt regular pangs of hunger, along with distracting yearnings for cookies, chips, and other low-quality foods. I would give in to those impulses at times and then quickly regret it. I was maintaining my weight, but I was not feeling in control of my body. I had worked hard on my personal development and extracted myself from a bad, self-destructive relationship. I now had a loving wife and a new baby. Here, too, though, my inner self told a starkly different story. I was not at peace. All my life I had wrestled with loneliness and had made some progress. Even in my seemingly idyllic circumstances, that sense of emptiness was always lurking.

At the time I was managing my life, but that was not enough. What I was searching for was a path to becoming *bulletproof*—to finding the unshakable inner strength that would let me become the master of all that I am, including the cravings for things that weren't good for me. (The idea of becoming bulletproof later inspired my book and my company of the same name.) That search was what brought me to the shaman. I wanted to confront true hunger, to the point where I could free myself from food and all the ways it occupied my mind. There's no way to fail at fasting if you're alone in the desert! I also wanted to work through my loneliness by facing down the kind of isolation that comes only by completely removing yourself from human contact.

So I walked into a cave in the Arizona desert and away from the rest of the world. For four solitary days I consumed only water and maybe a little Sonoran dust. By the time I walked back out, I had experienced a fast that changed my life. By reading this book, you have just taken the first step toward changing yours, too.

The needs that drove me to my journey were unique to me, but they were also rooted in the kinds of universal human challenges that we all face. In my case, I grew up as a fat kid. I eventually learned that I had been exposed to toxic mold that triggered Hashimoto's thyroiditis, a condition in which the body's immune system attacks the thyroid, but I didn't find that out until I was in my twenties. All I knew at the time was that I didn't look like the kids I admired; with my teenage man boobs, I certainly didn't look the way I wanted to.

If you struggle with your weight, and especially if you struggled with your weight when you were young, it's hard not to feel judged by other people. Add to that some early childhood trauma or schoolyard bullying, and there may be a part of you that always feels alone. A common coping mechanism is to develop an emotional addiction to food, to rely on eating to soothe the hard feelings. I say all this without a trace of self-pity, because I know that everyone who reads this book has gone through his or her own versions of these struggles, even if he or she has never been overweight. Almost everyone has some form of physical or psychological addiction to food. Maybe yours is candy. Maybe it's beer. Maybe it's bread and cheese; gluten and milk protein are both highly addictive. Or perhaps you're hooked on potatoes. Do you find it impossible to imagine life without French fries? I've been there.

The point is, addictions and cravings are built into us, even if you've never had a problem with your weight. They are easily activated, and there is a trillion-dollar food industry—what I call Big Food—that is specifically designed to do just that. When you're bored, you eat. When you're feeling stressed, you eat. Millions of years of evolutionary selection have hardwired us with these responses, as fundamental as our fear that things with sharp teeth might try to eat us. I sometimes refer to the four F's of survival: fear, food, the F-word that involves reproduction, and friends. Without food, you would never get to enjoy those last two F's, which is why the thought of going without food triggers such an intense, deeply irrational reaction before you even have time to think about it.

All of those thoughts were going through my head back in 2008 as I greeted the shaman and steeled myself for what lay ahead. Without being aware of it, I believed that even a single day without eating could leave me helplessly out of energy, which made me a prisoner to food. Going four days without food seemed a biological impossibility. This is how almost everyone in today's society thinks. You can bet that if you ask ten people what would happen to them if they didn't eat for a day or two, nine of them will say, "I'd starve." They even believe those words.

By the time I emerged from the cave, I'd started to realize that none of this is true. I came to recognize that there's a fundamental difference between hunger and craving. Hunger is a biological message, and it is something that you can control. Craving is a psychological need, and it is something that tries to control you. The truth is, you can go a long time without eating, and you won't suffer for it. In fact, you will thrive.

The Big Food industry has worked hard to convince you that craving and hunger are one and the same. If every craving means that you're about to starve, then you need to buy something to satisfy that craving immediately, right? And by a wonderful coincidence, Big Food is ready to take care of you with a candy bar that "really satisfies" and a thousand other processed drinks and snacks that shackle you to a relentless feeling of craving that subsides when you snack but never really leaves. The same dynamic plays out over and over every day, fooling us into thinking that we are prisoners to food. I wrote this book to help set you free and because no one wrote it for me when I was twenty-two and wearing size-46 pants.

GAIN WITHOUT PAIN

The key to that freedom is fasting—and learning how to do all styles of fasting without feeling pain, all the way from meal-skipping intermittent fasting to multiday fasts. What you'll learn here contradicts almost everything people think about what fasting is and what it does. Intermittent fasting won't make you weak, and it won't cause you to starve. It also doesn't require any one particular diet or one particular schedule of fasting, although you will experience a lot fewer cravings with some diets. Fasting is a tool kit that helps you unlock biological resources hidden in your body, resources you probably never knew you had.

Fasting can make you stronger and healthier, both physically and psychologically, by breaking you out of your food prison. It will free you from the burden of other people's opinions about how you should feel and even of how your body is telling you to feel. Ultimately, it will help you live your best life—to be your best self, putting the most out into the world.

I know these are extravagant-sounding claims, but they are supported by an abundance of scientific research, ancient wisdom practiced for millennia on every continent, and by many years of my own experimentation. Our palette of fasting options has expanded greatly in that time. I've tried various kinds of fasts, and I will share my findings with you. But the most important message that you're going to get from reading this book is just this: You can break away from the visceral feeling that if you skip a meal, or even several meals, you will be in danger—that you will be weak and miserable, unable to go on. You can overcome the feelings of fear, discomfort, starvation, terror, and loneliness, and replace them with liberation, power, and self-control. Work with me, and together we will make a better you. That matters more than whether you fast for a certain length of time or not.

Some of the things you want to change about yourself may be easy to spot. If you can't see your feet when you look down or notice a muffin top when you look to the side, your metabolism is broken, and we can fix that. Other issues are subtler: maybe you don't have the kind of energy and mental focus you wish you had. How many times a day do you catch yourself thinking about lunch instead of the meeting you're in? Fasting can help you with that, too. Then there are the most insidious problems—the ones so ubiquitous that you hardly notice them at all. Even if you look and feel fit, you probably live with a background hum of fear. There is an ancient part of you that is always worried about what will happen if your food goes away, and, by extension, you fear all of the other things that might go missing. It is a subtle, pervasive, biological survival instinct, but you don't have to let it control you.

All the way down at the cellular level, your body is programmed to think, "No matter how you're eating—what kinds of foods, how often, how much—I can't be sure what I'm getting will always be enough. Better store some extra." That relentless message cultivates a broader mindset of anxiety toward all kinds of other needs in your life, emotional as well as physical. Training yourself to confront your anxieties (about food or other things) and master them may be the greatest fasting benefit of all.

In this book, you will learn the methods of intermittent fasting, but I will also help you understand the tremendous scope of what fasting can do to you and for you. You're not ever going to choose to fast if you don't know why it matters. And you're definitely not going to choose to do it and stick with it if you associate fasting with suffering, misery, and deprivation.

When I came out of the shaman's cave, I felt great. That was when I realized that fasting doesn't need to be painful. It doesn't need to be hard. It's actually one of the most natural things you can do, because it is something that our species has naturally evolved to do. Fasting is a fundamental part of being human. After you finish this book and try some of these techniques until you find one that works for you, I am 100 percent convinced that you will like your life better than you did before—no matter what kind of diet you follow now, no matter what kinds of food you like to eat.

Remember what I said about intermittent fasting being a *tool kit*? I meant just that. It's not a single set of rules but an entire program for hacking your biology to make it work better. You can still eat the standard garbage diet of fast foods every day, if that's really what you want to do. You can be vegetarian, vegan, keto, Bulletproof, or anything else under the sun. Whatever type of diet you choose, if you eat your way in combination with the fasting techniques that I will describe here, you will be better off.

Here's another big surprise: you won't be hungry. Exactly the opposite. Intermittent fasting will set you free from hunger and all of the emotional baggage that comes with it.

Hunger heightens all your anxieties because it activates a powerful biochemical cascade in your brain. A lot of that action centers on a primitive brain structure known as the amygdala, which is about the size and shape of a small almond. That little structure is part of what Yale University neuroscientist Paul MacLean called the "reptilian brain"[1] because of its primal nature. The amygdala handles rapid, automatic emotional decisions that help keep you alive when you're not paying attention. It is the home of the "fight-or-flight" response that tells you to run away from a sudden lion attack or (more commonly these days) pull your hand away from a hot stove before you get burned. It can also trigger frightening spikes of hunger to make sure the body gets enough food—or more than enough, as the case was for me.

The actions of the amygdala were vital for our ancient ancestors, and they still serve a vital purpose in modern life. But as essential as the amygdala may be, it can also be a source of irrational, destructive fear. It's a major contributor to that voice in your head that says you might just die if you do something you're afraid of—such as going on a job interview, ending a bad relationship, speaking in public, or simply skipping a few meals.

Intermittent fasting enables you to put the amygdala and the whole reptilian part of your brain in its place, so that you can be more fully human, more fully yourself, less burdened by your fears. When you start out, you might feel uncomfortable for a day or two. Then you will feel liberated. It's not even hard. All you have to do is question a whole set of false assumptions about food and fasting:

What if it were easy to skip a meal—or two or three?

What if all fasts could be created equal?

What if you could eat and fast at the same time and have a better fast as a result?

What if you could use sleep and exercise to trick your body into thinking you're fasting?

What if fasting could be personalized to your gender and your genes?

What if fasting could make you both physically and mentally stronger?

You can do all of these things. I'll show you how. You can master your willpower and be in charge of yourself, more than you ever have before. Let's go.

FASTING IS ONLY IN YOUR HEAD

To set off on a vision quest, tradition dictates that a shaman guide you. But how do you find a shaman? It would be great if I could tell you about a secret spiritual network, but the truth is, I tracked my shaman down by doing a Google search. In retrospect, it probably would have been smarter to seek out a personal referral or maybe do a background investigation before signing on for such a momentous rite of passage. What can I say? I was drawn to the experience, and I was feeling impulsive.

That's not to say the shaman didn't deliver, mind you. It's just that some of her methods were . . . unique.

By tradition, shamans are rare, gifted humans who have attained a higher level of consciousness, enabling them to make a deep connection to the spiritual realm. The word itself gives you a sense of the tremendously rich history behind the practice. *Shaman* comes from the word *sha'man*,[1] a spiritual figure among the Tungu people of Siberia. Keep pressing back in time, and you can trace the word all the way to *sramana-s*, a term for a Buddhist ascetic in ancient Sanskrit. Sanskrit! That goes back more than three thousand years, well before ancient Rome and Greece. Sanskrit was the language of many of the primary texts of Buddhism and Hinduism. Nobody knows when shamanic practice first began, but there were probably shamans around—and fasting—when the pigments on the first cave painting were still wet.

Although I may not have known much about this particular shaman, I was well aware that I was tapping into a primal, powerful aspect of the human experience. I grew up in New Mexico, where I was as likely to see a cultural ceremony performed by an indigenous tribe as I was to experience Western religion. Later, I experimented with altered states and immersed myself in different types of meditation. When I walked into that cave, the most important thing I brought with me was a lack of preconceptions and a willingness to stay curious. If you truly want to experience the world, you need to keep yourself open to new experiences, including ones that come from beyond your own cultural background. Just be sure to approach other cultures with understanding and with respect and ask permission. Respectful inquiry has worked for me in the jungles of South America, in monasteries in Tibet, and even in the caves of Sedona. A good shaman will tell you to get lost if you're not a good fit and won't feel bad about it, either.

It takes an extraordinary mix of training, abilities, and background to become a shaman, but it's easy for someone to claim he or she is one without doing the work. Ancient peoples chose their shamans by their ability to sense things that others couldn't and put them through rigorous, often dangerous, training for years. Shamanic knowledge was passed down from generation to generation through that rigorous apprenticeship. Most shamans must experience extreme personal adversity and overcome it before they can earn the authority to help others. The help I was seeking was only half formed in my mind back then. I wanted someone who could lead a vision quest with fasting, to reset my relationship with food and loneliness, but I was aware of my spiritual and emotional hungers as well.

And then I met Delilah (not her real name; I've hidden her identity to protect her privacy). She owned a small ranch populated with llamas and alpacas. In her backyard, she had a sweat lodge equipped with LED lighting and subwoofers so she could play mind-altering sounds while sweating. Delilah was eccentric, for sure, but I was seeking out a guide who could take me on a vision quest, and I had a sense that this powerful, enigmatic, tattooed woman could get me where I needed to go.

I'm calling Delilah eccentric, but I wouldn't blame you if by now you're thinking that maybe *I'm* a little eccentric, too, for choosing a shaman instead of a therapist or for heading off into a cave in the middle of nowhere guided by a woman I'd never met before. It does seem a little out of the ordinary to seek inner peace this way—except that it's not. Whether it's to mark the end of childhood, to celebrate a religious holiday, to take a spiritual retreat, or simply to escape from the bustle of everyday life into the calm of nature, people will often travel to an isolated location in search of a life-altering experience. These outings commonly include fasting or other ways of breaking with routine. People do it in all walks of life, all around the world, and they regularly return a lot better than when they left.

Put more bluntly: We are all eccentric in our own superficial ways, yet we are all profoundly the same. We each seek our own, idiosyncratic path toward the same goals of controlling our hungers and overcoming our cravings, cravings for anything we want but don't have. That is exactly what makes fasting so powerful. Unlike many diets (or even some specific fasting plans you might have heard about), the program of fasting I'm talking about is not one rigid set of rules designed for one kind of person. It is a universal process of self-improvement that applies in specific, individual ways to every single person, based on biology, psychology, and even spirituality. It's more than what's (not) on your plate.

A LONG MENU OF FASTING OPTIONS

To understand what fasting does, let's begin with a clear picture of what fasting is. People use the term in many different ways, so we'll start by breaking it down to its essence. Its meaning is just two simple words: *going without.*

Note that I didn't say "going without food," because there are many ways to go without:

Sobriety is going without substances.

Meditation is going without thinking.

Solitude is going without other humans.

Sabbath (or Shabbat) is going without working.

Abstinence is going without sex and sexual release.

All of these are forms of fasting. They all involve turning away from something that people routinely feel they cannot live without. I know plenty of guys who say that they feel as though they're going to die if they go too long without an orgasm. Or maybe it's porn, a glass of wine, a piece of chocolate, or a busy day of feeling useful at the office. It may even be something that doesn't seem like an addiction at all, such as going to the gym. Whatever it is you think you need, fasting is about deciding that you are in charge of it—about summoning the internal fire to say "no."

I did many different forms of fasting in that cave, all at the same time. That's why it was scary. When you *go without*, it creates space in your mind to examine the things you think you depend on and to discover whether that dependence is truly what you thought it was. For instance, our dependence on oxygen is real . . . but most people freak out when their lungs are empty after about ten seconds, even though they know that they can go one or two minutes without oxygen. You can actually fast from oxygen. It's called hypoxic training, and it can increase endurance. Athletes often train[2] in high-altitude locations such as my hometown of Albuquerque, New Mexico, or Chamonix, France, to experience the benefits of doing with less oxygen, and the most powerful are now exposing themselves to brief periods of no oxygen, which drives superhuman biological changes. There are also ways to "fast" from oxygen by controlling your breathing, which can greatly enhance a meditative state; you'll learn more about that in chapter 7.

The same is true of food and drink: we do need those things, but we *think* we need them way before we actually do. (That goes for sex, companionship, work, and many other things, as well.) Examining your actual needs versus your perceived needs up close exposes how much power you actually have over your body and your behavior. You don't need to go into a cave to do that kind of self-evaluation. You can just carve out the quiet time to cross-examine your internal story about the things you are certain you can't do without. You will quickly discover that your certainties are not based on reality. Fasting from food, for instance, teaches you that you really don't need French fries. Each little step helps set you free.

While we're discussing what fasting is, I also want to clarify what fasting is not. *It is not suffering.* Although you may be uncomfortable the first few times you do it, fasting eventually becomes joyous and then transitions to . . . nothing consequential at all. Once you discover that you can do without, you gain power and control. When you end a fast from anything, it makes that substance or that experience much more appreciated. It causes heightened pleasure and brings easy gratitude into your life.

My ten-year-old son, inspired by the things he watched me do in the course of writing this book, recently decided he would try his own twenty-four-hour fast, with only a little black coffee in the morning. He was determined to pull it off, and he did. He turned down the fasting hacks you will learn about here, because he wanted to see what it was like to go it alone. At the end, he said, "Daddy, you're right. Fasting really is the best spice. That food I had for dinner was the best-tasting meal I've ever had!" Seeing the immense look of accomplishment and self-confidence in his smile made the father in me happy. My son felt that way because fasting puts you in control of the things you thought you couldn't live without. Fasting creates gratitude for things you probably took for granted. It's that simple—and that complicated.

There's another part of the definition that is absolutely crucial for you to know. *Fasting does not mean eliminating something from your life completely.* When athletes are hypoxic training, they are limiting their access to oxygen in a carefully controlled way; an uncontrolled oxygen fast is called suffocation. Even the most devout observer of the Sabbath will leap into action if he or she sees that someone is injured, because there are reasonable and unreasonable ways to give up work.

So it is with dietary fasting. We normally think of fasting to mean going without food entirely, but it is much more flexible than that. Fasting, in all of its forms, is most effective if it is responsive to your circumstances. An uncontrolled fast from food is simply starvation.

Which brings us to a final, crucial part of the definition. *Fasting is not just one thing.* There are many forms of dietary fasting. Have you ever heard of a dry fast? That's when you go without food and water. Have you ever heard of a dopamine fast?[3] My friend Cameron Sepah, a psychologist at the University of California San Francisco, created that concept. A dopamine fast is basically a break from all the instant gratification stimuli in your life, from shopping to gaming to alcohol and drugs. Or have you heard of people who go into a cave and stay there for a week or two in absolute darkness? That is fasting, too, from food and even light. Anytime you reduce the inputs to your body, you may be fasting.

I've been fasting regularly for more than ten years. Through a lot of wide-ranging research and experimentation I've found that the best way to fast regularly—no matter what you're going without—is a method called *intermittent fasting*.[4] It delivers remarkable benefits to your body and your mind. It is surprisingly easy to do, because it can be customized to the way you eat now, improving your life no matter what your style. It also painlessly opens the door to longer fasts.

The basic principle of intermittent fasting is that you toggle between short periods of doing without and periods of returning to your baseline behavior. This idea has been catching on lately, so you may have seen books and articles promoting specific ideas about the right way to do intermittent fasting. Some people cite scientific research in support of the so-called 16:8 intermittent fast, built around sixteen hours of going without. Others argue that an eighteen-hour fast might be somewhat better. Or twenty-four hours, based on yet another study. Then there are fasting-mimicking diets, in which you're allowed to eat so long as you limit yourself to a careful selection of foods, like the ones outlined in my Bulletproof Diet. A fast that includes food may sound like an oxymoron, but it's a real thing and it works. It's an important part of the fasting tool kit. I'll explain more about that later.

The bottom line is, there's no clear-cut rule of how long those "periods without" need to be, as long as they give you what you seek. In fact, obsessing over the rules runs counter to the big-picture goals of what fasting is supposed to achieve. We can therefore stop focusing on the details of the fast and instead pay attention to the shape of what fasting does for you. The details are just that: details.

HOW FASTING HACKS THE BODY

So what does fasting do for you?

One significant benefit is that *fasting regulates your insulin levels.* After you eat, your body breaks down carbohydrates from food into a sugar called glucose, which is one of the primary molecular energy sources in the body. The glucose level in your bloodstream goes up. In response, the pancreas secretes insulin, a hormone that acts as a kind of metabolic switch. The insulin attaches to cells in your body and causes them to fuel up on glucose. Finally, your body unleashes other hormones, including cholecystokinin and leptin, to signal that you're full and to convince you to stop eating.

That is how the system is supposed to work, but the modern Big Food diet can overwhelm those delicate biological mechanisms, which evolved in a world where bad fats didn't exist and honey was the only sweet thing available most of the year. Companies are under constant pressure to sell you the cheapest sources of calories, and those sources are almost always the least desirable from a health standpoint. To boost the appeal of those budget calories, the companies blend them with artificial flavors, artificial sweeteners, and whatever else they can to make the resulting product taste good. It's not as though there's anyone evil out there who wants you to be sick. These are just businesspeople doing what businesspeople do, trying to maximize profits and minimize costs. From the consumer's point of view, though, the lack of evil intent is beside the point. All that matters is the result: supermarket shelves jammed full of processed foods that are mismatched to human metabolism.

If you eat a processed diet full of refined sugar and low-cost carbs, your body can't always keep up with the flood of calories you're consuming. The ramped-up flavors and sweetness in processed foods also tend to scramble the digestive system's normal "stop-eating" signals, compounding the problem. When there is more energy coming into the body than there is going out, the extra glucose will be stored as fat. At the same time, your pancreas will be overworking in a frantic attempt to keep things in balance. Eventually your body may become insensitive to insulin; that's a leading cause of type 2 diabetes.

Fasting slows down this insulin-glucose cycle and gives your body a rest. Such a rest period is especially welcome if you are eating low-quality foods, which is why fasting benefits everyone regardless of his or her normal diet. Basically, consuming less of the bad stuff for even a brief period helps. While you're taking a break between meals, your body will also draw on its stored reserves of sugar and fat. Your glucose levels will remain stable, while your insulin levels will drop. Adrienne Barnosky, an endocrinologist at Duke University School of Medicine, and her colleagues confirmed that intermittent fasting helps prevent insulin resistance.[5] There is persuasive clinical evidence that fasting helps prevent leptin resistance as well, which matters because leptin resistance is the first step of insulin resistance. As long as you don't eat anything that raises your blood sugar, you can get most of the same benefits even while eating; that's the principle behind a fasting-mimicking diet.

Another benefit of fasting: *It triggers autophagy*, a self-cleaning (literally "self-eating") process in the body. Through the normal wear and tear of living, your cells gradually clog up with accumulated toxins, pathogens, misshapen proteins, and dead cell parts. All of that microscopic garbage can impair the normal operation of your cells, and can even make it so that they don't divide and reproduce correctly. Autophagy is a whole package of biomolecular tools that constantly sweep through the body, collect the trash, and deposit it into tiny digestive vessels called lysosomes.[6] Autophagy is essential for keeping your cells in good working order.

A growing number of studies indicate that triggering autophagy also helps slow the aging process, reduce inflammation, and enhance your body's performance overall. Researchers still don't totally understand why fasting boosts autophagy, and most of the studies have been done on mice, not on humans, but the biological mechanism seems to operate much the same way across the animal kingdom: when the body isn't busy moving sugar and storing fat, it devotes more resources to basic maintenance. One recent study at the Scripps Research Institute in La Jolla, California, found especially pronounced cleanup of the neurons in the brain during fasting.[7]

More and more studies are finding that *fasting makes your body work more efficiently and cleanly* at the molecular level, in a complex set of ways that we are still exploring. For instance, a group of Japanese biologists reported in 2019 that a fifty-eight-hour fast—in people, not in mice!—increased the blood levels of forty-four different compounds that are involved in the chemical pathways that break down fat and control the structures of proteins.[8]

Intermittent fasting has been shown to influence a potent anti-aging molecule known as nicotinamide adenine dinucleotide, or NAD. In its activated form, it's known as NAD+. The deceptively simple-sounding job of NAD+ is to shuttle electrons around so that the chemical reactions in your body can proceed smoothly. That little molecule works hard: it enables your cells to generate energy; it helps repair the damage to your DNA that happens all the time; it keeps your proteins properly shaped, which is key to avoiding mental decline; and it protects your cells from oxidative stress, one of the relentless processes at the heart of aging. Intermittent fasting increases the levels of NAD+ in your blood. Seriously, you want that.

Every time I think I've caught up with the literature on the biological benefits of fasting, something new catches my eye and surprises me. A recent study out of MIT[9] found that fasting for twenty-four hours substantially improves the ability of stem cells to regenerate. It appears to promote the growth of new nerve cells in your brain and to expand the brain's ability to adapt to stimuli. Fasting even does good work on your microbiome, the ecosystem of bacteria that live in your gut. When these bacteria are deprived of food, they secrete a hormone called fasting-induced adipose factor; this hormone instructs the body to stop storing fat and start burning it instead.

In almost every instance, these fasting benefits don't require going without food entirely. In 2014, I wrote about a special kind of intermittent fasting created to make it painless to ease into intermittent fasting.[10] It led, in large part, to all the people who used it collectively losing an estimated 1 million pounds. It's similar to 16:8 fasting but with a key difference: In the morning, while you're taking a break from solid food, you drink a cup of Bulletproof Coffee, which contains fats that help people not feel hungry while they're going without the stuff that they usually eat but keep insulin and protein metabolism silent. "Butter MCT coffee intermittent fasting" sounded silly, so I named it Bulletproof Intermittent Fasting a decade ago. Because it works, it has stood the test of time, and there are hundreds of thousands of views of the videos I've done about it.

With this version of intermittent fasting, the type of fats that you consume matters. Corn oil, soybean oil, canola oil, and seed oils contain unstable fats that can contribute to inflammation and other undesirable effects. Grass-fed butter and MCT oil are much healthier. (MCT stands for medium-chain triglyceride, a group of fatty molecules that are relatively small and therefore easy for the body to absorb and process for energy.) These are the types of fats that go into Bulletproof Coffee, and they have been staples of my diet for the past decade.

Bulletproof Intermittent Fasting is a way to turn on the insulin-stabilizing and autophagy benefits of fasting while managing the other, less pleasant biological effects of fasting. I'm talking, of course, about the hungry/hangry feeling you get, especially when you are new to the fast and haven't yet adapted to it. That's the reptilian part of your brain talking. You can either use a bunch of energy to struggle with it to remain in control or tell it to shut the hell up with a cup of creamy coffee and save the energy for something better. Either way, your body thinks you fasted.

I suggest that you start fasting in the way I have developed through much research and trial—a way that works for almost everyone. Wake up in the morning and drink a cup of Bulletproof Coffee: black coffee, a dollop of grass-fed butter, and a teaspoon or more of C8 MCT oil. It's the best latte you'll ever drink. C8 MCT oil is a flavorless extract of coconut oil that has the ability to suppress hunger and increase energy in your body. The quality fats will keep you full until lunchtime. At the molecular level, you will continue autophagy and fat burning. At the personal level, you won't miss your familiar breakfast at all. Instead of using up precious willpower to fight back against your hunger response, you are biologically pressing the "off" button on your food cravings.

Bulletproof Coffee hacks the feeling of hunger during fasting by boosting the level of *ketones* in your blood. Ketones are another important part of the biology of fasting. If your body isn't getting enough glucose from what you're eating and drinking, your liver and muscles use all the carbohydrates stored in your body, then prepare an alternate source of energy by converting fat into smaller molecules— ketones. The ketones circulate through the bloodstream and go to your muscle cells and other body tissues. This state is called ketosis; your body is literally burning fat as its primary fuel source.

Ketones not only provide energy, they also make you more alert. I recently met with Satchidananda Panda, an expert on the body's internal circadian rhythm clock, as he was working at the Salk Institute in La Jolla, California. As we walked down the central outdoor path at the institute, I could see why its architect created it to be "worthy of a visit by Picasso." Even so, Satchin's research is far more epic than the buildings. He's found that ketones act as miniature alarm bells, rousing the brain cells that regulate the circadian rhythm and instructing the body to switch into an active, awake state.[11] A small rise in ketones from fasting provides a burst of energy, which likely evolved to help you have a more successful hunt. It is an evolutionary gift from our ancestors, and you can turn on that burst of energy at will by using ketosis. Ketones in the morning, when you "break fast," flip the switch on that energy for many hours.

C8 MCT oil is converted directly into ketones in the body, and coffee contains caffeine, which doubles your ketone production, according to a study by Canadian researchers.[12] An elevated ketone level stimulates production of cholecystokinin, or CCK (the "stop eating" hormone) and cuts off production of another troublemaking hormone, ghrelin, which is produced in the stomach and small intestine. Biologists have nicknamed ghrelin the "hunger hormone" because it stimulates the desire to eat and activates the hypothalamus, a part of the brain that helps regulate appetite. It's all part of the many overlapping, synergistic benefits of intermittent fasting.

These days, people often use a term I created a decade ago, *biohacking*, to describe fine-tuning your control of your body. That word makes it sound like a futuristic idea, which is only half true. Adjusting the way you eat to promote healing and wellness is an ancient practice—as ancient as life itself. The biological mechanisms for self-cleansing and rejuvenation have been built into us by billions of years of evolution, as have our instinctive responses to food. What's new is that we can study the processes happening inside us at the molecular level; understand exactly why they are happening; and make deliberate choices to enlist those processes for maximum benefit with minimum discomfort.

FAST YOUR WAY

Depending on your current lifestyle, fasting might put your body through some significant changes. I therefore recommend that you start gently, which will minimize any initial discomfort and bring you more quickly to the joyous stages of fasting. You might start your day with coffee and a teaspoon or two of MCT oil. Hey, maybe you're a big guy and you need more. You read this and think, "I'm 400 pounds, and there's no way I'm going to survive on a couple tiny teaspoons of MCT." Fine, use a tablespoon or more if your body tells you it needs more. You can even try switching to black coffee some days and see if you feel better or more alert. The specifications are up to you; what matters is that your biological systems are going to read the chemistry in your blood and determine that you're fasting even though you're drinking a cup of coffee and don't feel hungry.

It's not just a fake-out. Contrary to what water-drinking pedantic fasters might suggest, you're really fasting! You're fasting because you aren't eating any protein, so your body doesn't need to use up any of its protein-digesting molecules (proteases) to break down food, and your insulin level doesn't change. Instead, your body is devoting all of those resources to folding new proteins, cleaning up old cells, and repairing cellular damage—that is, it's busy doing autophagy. Though you think you're eating, your body thinks it's fasting. All the right healing mechanisms are already there in your body; all you have to do is set them free to do their job unhindered.

Maybe the idea of replacing breakfast with a coffee concoction just doesn't sound great to you. At least it's far better tasting than a kale smoothie, which doesn't taste good and isn't good for you, either. There's still a way to get the benefits of fasting: try a *protein fast*. Protein fasting means that one day a week, or longer, you eat less than 15 grams of protein from all sources, including vegetables. You can enjoy some fat, have some vegetables (just not high-protein vegetables such as lima beans and spinach), and eat almost anything that's not high protein or straight sugar. Do that once a week, and you're going to get many of the benefits of fasting without fasting, because a low protein intake lowers insulin and a critical metabolic protein called mTOR,[13] exactly as fasting does. As I said: fasting is going without, but going without doesn't always mean going without *everything*. You get to pick.

This kind of flexibility is sure to piss off the fasting purists. There are some people out there who love ironclad rules for how to live your life. I'm sure you've met a lot of them or at least seen their comments online. There are people who genuinely believe that they aren't dieting or fasting correctly unless they're suffering. That's not my fast. I'm going to do what works, even if there are no studies yet showing *why* it works. I've used protein fasting for more than a decade, and I've spoken to many other people who've adopted it since I set out the basic principles in my book *The Bulletproof Diet*. So I can tell you: protein fasts work; simple as that.

If you can't live without protein, you can try another kind of fasting: don't eat carbs; ingest only fat and protein. There's a name for that kind of fasting, and it's all the rage: the keto diet. What if we add onto that? How about avoiding inflammatory proteins and inflammatory fats? Your diet may be chock full of inflammatory fats without your knowing it, since Big Food doesn't tell you (and often doesn't even know) which fats are harmful to you. Many common oils—including canola, corn, peanut, and soybean—are inflammatory omega-6 fats. You may be amazed how much better you'll feel if you get rid of them.

Plus, gluten and casein (milk protein) are inflammatory, and you won't get results if those are your protein sources. All of these different approaches fall within the scope of Bulletproof Intermittent Fasting. We'll discuss even more ways to fast in chapter 10.

Close your eyes for a moment, and picture what you imagined a fast would look or feel like before you started reading this book. Perhaps you were picturing a health fanatic exerting some sort of Herculean effort to refuse all food—and yourself suffering in an attempt to emulate that effort. I don't blame you; there are plenty of books, magazines, and infomercials promoting this stereotype. Now close your eyes again, grab hold of those images, and erase them from your mind. I want to prepare you for embracing a fasting method designed around *selectively and surgically going without.* I want you to learn how to fast in any way that works for you—not just this week or this month or even this year but for the rest of your life. Fasting has to be sustainable to be meaningful, and being sustainable means that you make the least possible effort and feel the least possible pain.

You read that right: the least possible effort; the least possible pain.

Your decision to travel down this path will lead you into a very different world. You're going to unleash the power of all of those biological mechanisms in your cells. They've been honed by millions of years of natural selection to take care of you. You just have to learn how to activate them correctly—to make them work for you, rather than the other way around.

Unlike other methods of fasting or dieting, I promise that when you *fast this way* you won't be hungry. You won't be cold, you won't be tired, you won't have brain fog, you won't be hangry, you won't be hypogly-bitchy (that's the foul mood that often strikes when you have low blood sugar, or hypoglycemia). The ketones and metabolites and NAD+ and leptin and all of the other biochemicals you are enlisting will take care of you. You'll feel focused at work all day and come home in a good mood. Your brain will feel sharper than ever and you'll feel younger, with a gut that will repair itself. You'll lose weight, too, even though that's not the primary goal of intermittent fasting. What matters the most is that you'll have the energy and clarity to pursue whatever it is that you want in life.

Your entry into the world of fasting begins the same as my entry into the shaman's cave: you push ahead, take the first step, then another. Put it to your own personal test. Try going for twenty-four hours on just water and see how you like that. Or maybe try experimenting with just water and then black coffee in the morning. Don't eat anything on the second day until two in the afternoon and see how you like that. If you're metabolically fit, your body digests fat well, and you're used to fasting, it's not going to matter. You'll be just fine. But if you're new to this, and you are like I used to be in my twenties, you're going to feel like crap on just water or black coffee. Anxiety. Anger. Brain fog. That's fine, too. It will get easier with time, or you can explore a whole range of intermittent fasting biohacks here that make it easier *now*. Experimentation is part of the fun, as you learn more about yourself. Again, suffering is not the goal.

There's another hack you should know in order to fast like a boss. Sometimes you'll take on a fast because there's something bad going on in your gut. You know what I'm talking about: there's rumbling, there are things no one wants to smell, and, well, you have a most inconvenient problem. The best solution is to not have anything inside your gut, which will suppress the bad behavior of your internal bacteria. When your gut bacteria don't have any food, they freak out. In fact, they freak out so badly that they make something called FIAF— fasting induced adipose factor—which they use to sneakily tell your body to burn extra fat for energy, so the bacteria's home (your gut) will stay alive longer. This works to your advantage, except that when gut bacteria get stressed, they also increase the production of a group of compounds called lipopolysaccharides. And let me tell you, when lipopolysaccharides come across your gut barrier, you are not going to like how you feel. They are well-known toxins. This is one of the reasons that when you first go into ketosis or first start fasting, you typically get what is known as "keto flu."

One of the simplest hacks is adding a little activated charcoal to your fasting protocol. It binds directly to those lipopolysaccharide molecules, which is probably why ingestion of activated charcoal extends animal (and likely human) life span,[14] but it doesn't stop the good guy, FIAF, according to current research. Taking activated charcoal is also a simple way to help soothe the gut pain and many other discomforts that might occur when you first start fasting. I've been sharing the benefits of activated charcoal for years, but it's hardly original with me; it was a part of indigenous American dietary traditions for unknown ages before Europeans arrived. Various Native American peoples knew that activated charcoal soaks up toxins in the gut and tames the production of intestinal gas. I found it in the jungles of Peru and in Nepal; it's one of the earliest remedies known to humans. It works even when you're not fasting but are just experiencing a stomachache.

While you are taking control of your internal biology through fasting, you also want to take control of your microbiome. Collectively, there are about as many bacteria in your body as there are human cells. According to the latest estimate coming out of the Weizmann Institute of Science in Israel, there are about 30 trillion of them living inside you![15] They are much more than microbial hitchhikers; they are an integral part of your internal ecosystem, to the extent that some medical scientists now call the microbiome a "supporting organ." Your gut bacteria help break down complex carbohydrates, neutralize toxic compounds, aid in the synthesis of certain amino acids and vitamins (including B-complex vitamins), and produce compounds that influence your metabolism.

The vast majority of your microbiome should be helpful or at least benign, but there are some bad actors mixed in there, too. In a well-balanced microbiome, the good bacteria help keep the harmful ones in check. For all these reasons, you want to take antibiotics only as a last resort. Many antibiotic drugs are "broad spectrum," meaning that they slaughter both good and bad bacteria indiscriminately. It's like burning down an old forest, full of a rich diversity of wildlife, to get rid of a patch of poison ivy. Your microbiome will bounce back once you finish your course of medication, but it probably won't be quite the same as before—and there's a chance that you will have created more opportunity for the bad bacteria by clearing out so many of the good ones.

When you're fasting, you need to keep the health of your microbiome in mind. This is a fairly new concept. Although people have long understood the importance of maintaining a healthy gut, it's only in the past decade or so that scientists have begun to decode[16] the vast number of intricate, intimate biochemical interactions between you and your microbes. With that knowledge now in hand, we can begin to expand the concept of biohacking to include hacking your microbiome during fasting.

Some ecosystems require an occasional drought or fire to clear out old brush and allow new seeds to sprout. Your gut biome will almost certainly benefit from an occasional longer fast for the same reasons, and fasting can eliminate bad bacteria in the gut. The problem is that excessive fasting can also knock out good gut bacteria, and most of us don't get enough fiber to feed the good guys anyway.

To maintain healthy gut bacteria levels with or without a fast, you can take various types of prebiotic fiber. These are marvelously useful substances that are compatible with most kinds of fasts. Soluble fiber attracts water in your stomach and intestines and turns into a gel, which slows the digestive process. Common sources of dietary fiber include oats, bran, nuts, and seeds, none of which are fasting compatible. Instead, you can opt for a blend of acacia gum, guar gum, and larch arabinogalactan. These scary-sounding things are just plant-based tree saps that you can buy as flavorless powders that blend well into coffee or any other liquid.

Technically, these prebiotic fibers are carbohydrates, but the fibers are a tough form of carbohydrate that cannot be digested and burned as carbs by your body. Instead, they become a food source for your microbiome, which breaks the fibers into ketogenic fats. Those fats act to switch off the sensation of hunger during your fast, while the bulking properties of the fiber make you feel full. Pretty clever biohack, right?

When you take prebiotic fibers, you get none of the carbohydrate effects that you would normally get, but your levels of good bacteria explode. These fibers are shown to increase your life span and reduce all-cause mortality. Prebiotic fibers moderate the changes in your blood sugar, adding to the insulin-regulating benefits of fasting. Here's the kicker: these fibers are also associated with weight loss. If you take soluble fiber while you fast, you don't get a complete gut rest, but you do get all the energy benefits and all the longevity benefits, and you don't feel the pain of the fast. It's almost impossible to be hungry after mixing 20 grams of prebiotic fiber and a little MCT into a cup of black coffee.

Most ancient fasting practices also involve drinking at least a little bit of tea. As you know, I prefer coffee in my modern fast. Why? Well, the amount of caffeine in two small cups of coffee will double your ketone production, and ketones are what you want when you're fasting. Coffee and fasting go together like motherhood and apple pie or teenagers and cell phones. I strongly recommend coffee in the morning (and not just because I created Bulletproof Coffee!). It really does make a difference. If you're not a particular fan of drinking coffee, think of it as the fasting equivalent of eating kale. You may not like the taste of kale, but you eat it because you've been programmed to believe it's such a healthy food. Look at coffee as a superfood for your fast, another part of the tool kit that allows you to direct the way your biology works.

You've now learned about three remarkable and remarkably simple components of an effective fast: coffee, MCT oil, and soluble fiber. All of them will enable you to turn off hunger, take in calories, and still maintain your fast. Maybe you didn't believe me before when I told you that fasting is not about suffering? I hope you're starting to believe now.

You may hear people say that if you're consuming caffeine, fats, and fiber (even small amounts), you are not technically fasting. Generally speaking, those people are either purists trying to justify their own pain, or they are trying to sell you something. Over the years, hundreds of thousands of people have looked into my work on intermittent fasting—everyone from research scientists to the engaged readers of my books and blog. They can all testify that it works. I can also confirm that personally, as someone who has lost weight and kept it off and who has routinely practiced intermittent fasting for years. Best of all, you don't have to take any of this on faith. You can run the experiment on yourself and quickly discover firsthand that this approach really works.

If you're into self-flagellation, feel free to grit out your fast without these biohacks. Just be prepared to endure the kind of needless pain that will get in the way of the rest of your life as your metabolism becomes stronger. Think about running a business, finding a new job, or tending to a kid hanging off each arm. Do you want to face those challenges feeling hungry, weak, and irritable as your body adapts? Or do you want to come at them from a place of strength, peace, and vigor?

When you fast this way, you fast *your* way. The biochemical systems in your body determine how your body responds to fasting, but you determine how to activate them. You are in control of what fasting does to you. *The most important thing fasting does to you is that it puts you in charge of your life.*

What Does Fasting Do for You?

- Makes your body burn fat (ketosis)

- Helps your gut heal itself

- Provokes the body's self-cleaning (autophagy) and detoxification processes

- Reduces your risk of almost every chronic disease

- Causes your body to produce more stem cells

- Reduces your risk of type 2 diabetes by improving insulin sensitivity

- Slows aging from oxidative stress

- Reduces inflammation—both brain inflammation and love handles

- Boosts your emotional state, building self-confidence

- Improves your relationship with food

- Enhances your ability to enter a spiritual and meditational state

OTHER WAYS OF *GOING WITHOUT*

I've been talking mostly about the effects of fasting from food, but remember that there are many other types of fasting. Maybe you want to cut back on alcohol, for instance. The same principles apply. This is not an all-or-nothing situation, unless you're an alcoholic—in which case I encourage you to find the support you need to get healthy. Going without alcohol for thirty, sixty, or ninety days is an alcohol fast. You're not giving it up, you're just *going without* for a while. Alcohol fasting provides significant benefits, including a reduction in liver fat, less inflammation, and dramatically better sleep. It helps detoxify the liver and pancreas, strengthens the heart, and sharpens the communication pathways in the brain.[17] Although I really want to believe the claims that moderate drinking is harmless and may even have some health benefits, the science just doesn't support this wishful thinking. Alcohol disrupts certain neural pathways in the brain. It stresses the liver and promotes the production of toxins in the pancreas. It carries lipopolysaccharides into your blood. It increases your risk of several types of cancer, including liver and esophageal cancer. It can lead to heart arrhythmias and cardiomyopathy, a stiffening of the heart muscle. So yes, alcohol fasting is a good thing.

Or maybe you decide you want to fast from tobacco. I don't have to tell you about the benefits of quitting cigarettes, because they should be obvious even if you're a smoker. Treating your break from tobacco as a fast can make it easier to break free from it entirely. A central part of fasting is telling your body that there will be brief periods where you don't get the things you feel you need. With tobacco this is a particular challenge, because it is a highly addictive substance, especially because cigarettes contain nontobacco flavoring agents that dramatically increase addiction. But you know what? Food is addictive, too, yet you can learn to master it. Remember the difference between a craving and a hunger: when your body tells you that you *need* something like a cigarette, it's lying to you. Smoking is a powerful craving, but it is a craving all the same. It is something the body wants but not something it needs. And despite all the stories, nicotine withdrawal peaks on the third day after you quit.[18] After that, it's about understanding why you choose to do what you do.

But go in with your eyes open. You are messing with powerful forces inside your body and mind, and they may not give up easily. They certainly did a number on me during my vision quest in the cave. A certain amount of discomfort is normal when you begin to confront those wants. Whether it's food or alcohol or a cigarette, your body may seem to be screaming at you that it needs the thing you are taking away. Develop the discipline to silence the screams. Don't assume you can simply think your way through this. You can sail through it with the biohacks that make fasting easier, regardless of what you are fasting from, or you can muscle your way through with willpower alone. Sleep, exercise, breathing, and meditation can all help. You'll read a lot more about them in the upcoming chapters.

It bears repeating, because it's such an essential idea, that the key to any successful fast is learning to feel safe when *going without*. The thing you are going without doesn't even need to be a substance. It can be a lifestyle or pattern of behavior. Many years ago, I was getting my MBA at Wharton while working full time, and I couldn't keep up with all the things I was doing. I realized I had to go on a media fast to save my sanity. I switched off the TV and stopped paying my cable bill so that I couldn't be tempted to turn it back on. I realized that I'd been putting so much time and energy into watching television that it was disrupting my ability to graduate—which I barely did anyway.

Once I got used to not watching TV, I realized how much I hadn't really wanted to watch it in the first place. Today, more than twenty years later, I've kept my TV-free habit. I've probably saved a few thousand dollars and definitely saved many thousands of hours of my time, time that I was able to use more productively. Instead of watching TV three or four hours a day, I've been reading books, writing, recording almost a thousand podcast episodes, starting companies, and playing with my kids. It all started with a planned two-year TV fast.

I certainly didn't think of it that way at the time, but I was doing a form of biohacking when I gave up TV. Just as Big Food caters to the dietary cravings in your brain, the entertainment industry has developed techniques to cater to sensory cravings in your brain. The sounds, rhythms, and storytelling techniques are designed to stir up dopamine in your brain. Eating junk food makes you feel safe, by design. Bingeing shows on Netflix or chewing through YouTube videos can also make you feel safe because they let you avoid the stressful thoughts and feelings circling around in your head. No wonder people indulged all of these things like mad during pandemic isolation. A certain amount of indulgence can be harmless, even essential, to staying sane during stressful times. The sense of safety can be an illusion, however. Occasional, helpful indulgences can become self-destructive coping strategies. At the very least, they are almost certainly diverting time and energy from other things that you want to do with your life.

That's why Cameron Sepah recommends dopamine fasting: to help break you free from those cravings. A dopamine fast helps liberate your brain from its addiction to the emotional jolts of movies and TV shows. When your body expends less energy on metabolizing junk food, it devotes more resources to autophagy and cellular repair. When your mind expends less energy processing junk culture, it devotes more resources to the creativity and original thinking.

That's why I also recommend that you try intermittent social media fasting. Believe me, I'm not saying social media is a bad thing. It keeps us connected to people we might never talk to otherwise; it has maintained and strengthened a lot of relationships in my life even as it stokes divisions in society and censors useful health information. But I'm going to make a wild guess that you spend more time on social media that you'd like to—and I'd bet I'm right, except that I don't gamble. Every text message, every Facebook post, every tweet scrolling by is another little dopamine hit in your brain. It's hard to resist.

The incremental, adaptable style of fasting works here, too. Try not picking up your phone until noon. An intermittent social media fast? You'll find that it's an amazing feeling—and much harder to do than you might think. What I did, and what I do to this day, is tie my social media with at least the beginning of my intermittent food fast. I leave my phone in airplane mode overnight, so when I wake up in the morning, I don't have any Internet content. I don't see any texts, and I don't have access to my social media accounts. My rule is that until I drop my kids off at school—or now that home schooling is a thing, until after I sit down with the kids while they eat breakfast—I'm on my intermittent social media fast. Two years ago, I began posting notices on my Instagram account to let my followers know when I'm media fasting. I was pleasantly surprised by how positively people responded. They supported the idea, and they respected my time when I went dark. You don't have to delete Facebook; just limit the window of time you allow yourself to look at it. You don't have to give up food, either; just limit when you eat it.

At first it felt odd to fast from social media. I didn't have any clever biohacks to help me out, no digital equivalent of MCT and fiber. It was more like the shock therapy of going into the cave. But soon I became more aware of my tendency to overuse my phone. Then media fasting started to become natural. Now if I pick up my phone to do work-related social media in the morning, it actually feels weird.

A wonderful paradox of fasting is that it can make you feel calmer. That just sounds wrong, doesn't it? How can you take away the things that make you feel safe and satisfied yet end up feeling *safer*? The secret is that fasting is a habit changer. You will go without something and realize you didn't actually need it. The fasting literally changes your body and reprograms your brain. It makes you stronger. It activates your innate energy generation and self-repair mechanisms, in all of their forms. The result is that you feel more self-confident, more self-sufficient, and simply better.

First you have to get started, though, and you're not going to get very far if your initial impression is that fasting is a difficult, miserable experience. That is why it's so important to master the art of having a cup of coffee and a little MCT oil or prebiotic fiber for breakfast. By using that hack and many others I'll tell you about in the coming chapters, you can skip the pain while getting all the benefits of fasting. At the same time that it makes you stronger, fasting opens up your awareness of who is in control of your body: you are! Once you assert more power over the way you eat, it will be much easier to assert similar power over how you use social media or how you confront any of the other unwanted cravings in your life.

Fasting is like a Swiss Army knife, an incredibly impactful tool that has far more use than just weight loss. Through fasting you realize the feeling of self-control, and self-control leads you to make better decisions about the air you breathe, the food you eat, and the content you consume.

Every action has a return on investment for it. In business, they call it ROI, shorthand for whether or not you are applying your resources in a smart way. Fasting has a very high ROI, whereas the return on investment from eating French fries is very low: a brief hit of dopamine from the salty goodness, followed by twenty-four hours of inflammation from the damaging fats. When you think about what fasting does for you on the cellular level and then consider what eating low-quality food does to you in comparison, it's obvious why this is true. The ROI on a glass of wine is better than the fries, but it is still negative if you look at how it destroys good sleep. Social media helps you stay connected with friends and know what's going on in the world, but it also allows you to be controlled by your favorite social media algorithm. With every craving, think about whether you're getting a good ROI. If you're not, give it up for half a day, and see what happens.

Fasting allows you to think clearly about those choices, because it heightens your awareness. It puts you in control of your biology. It lets you make your own rules, which is a core part of being human. When I say make your own rules, that applies to everything—even to fasting itself. Throughout this book I'll share some of the fasting methods that have worked best for me, but don't forget who is really calling the shots: *you create your own fast.*

It's your life to do your way. Choose what you would like to do without, and then make it happen.

2

ENLISTING YOUR
MOLECULAR MACHINES

In retrospect, it seemed as though I had prepared all my adult life for a vision quest in a cave. Despite being the son of an engineer, from a family of hard-core scientists, I'd always been a closet seeker, reading spiritual literature and curiously exploring philosophies that weren't a natural fit for a rationalist like me. At first, my seeking was fueled by a burning desire to understand how people could believe in ideas that, to me, seemed ridiculous or impossible. I took so many religion courses in college that in my senior year, I discovered I was only one class away from accidentally earning a minor in religious studies. In one such seminar a wise professor asked the class what all of the world's most extreme and violent religious fanatics had in common. In my youthful arrogance, I said, "They're all irrational." His reply: "No. They are completely rational. They just have different beliefs and assumptions than you do, and they behave accordingly. Their actions are rational if you believe what they do."

Those words really set me on a new path, because I thought I was rational, but I had not tested most of my beliefs about the world. I had already learned that my assumptions about what to eat to stay thin were wrong, and I began to wonder whether how many of my other assumptions about the way the world worked were actually true.

In my early thirties I traveled to Tibet to study meditation with the local masters. I witnessed several sadhus, spiritual men who fasted for weeks as part of their ascetic lifestyle and practiced self-denial without dying—or suffering. I realized that my beliefs about what the human body could endure were too limiting. I started to become a guinea-pig kind of guy who would jump into any situation with both feet if I identified it as something that scared me. The more I did this, the more I realized that facing down your fears is liberating. I used to be afraid of heights, so I would go up to the top of tall buildings and lean over the edge until I conquered the fear. It was terrifying—until one day when it wasn't anymore. Was I fasting from a feeling of comfort at those times? Actually, yes. I didn't die even though it felt as if I would, and it made me stronger.

All of this is to say that over the years I've gotten comfortable with pushing my boundaries, especially when I think that doing so will result in personal growth. It was with all these experiences tucked away inside me that I filled out an online form to set up my vision quest, and then I talked to the shaman, Delilah, on the phone. Her personality definitely seemed a little extreme for my comfort level, and I could feel my skepticism and probably some fear creeping into our dialogue. Perfect! Already pushing my fear buttons. As we spoke, she shared the sorts of stories that sounded like the shamanic experiences I'd read about, experiences that were truly transformative. So I figured: this is a person who walks the talk. We agreed to work together, we set a date for my challenge, and I flew out to Arizona.

Delilah's ranch was located near Sedona, in the middle of a national forest. Sedona has some of the most spectacular landscapes on Earth. The soil there is a saturated red—in this case, the postcards don't lie—and everywhere you look you see strange spires and cliffs cut into the soft rock by ancient rivers and winds. Seen through the eyes of a desert native, the land was teeming with life among the sparse scrub. All around me I noticed spiny cactuses, venomous rattlesnakes, and lots of tiny birds, each uniquely adapted to the striking but harsh environment. The sky there is a different kind of blue, and the sunsets are a color that hasn't yet been named, not even in the extra-large box of crayons you coveted as a child.

When I showed up at Delilah's house, she fed me watermelon juice, which, it turns out, can stabilize blood glucose levels even though it has a high glycemic index, making it a useful way to initiate a fast. She reminded me that I was about to be dropped into the wilderness in the morning—as if I needed a reminder. One of the central goals of my vision quest was to endure intense solitude. In the back of my mind, I knew I was afraid of being alone. I was afraid of being hungry. I was afraid of not having something to eat when I felt lonely. It was time to bring all of these fears to the surface so I could face them head-on.

But even as I arrived for my solitary vision quest, the shaman greeted another seeker who showed up for the same spiritual journey. I was so pissed that I almost went home. You know that feeling when something you desperately wanted suddenly seems impossibly out of reach? Whether it was fear or true outrage talking, I still don't know. I just know that in the moment, it seemed as though my vision quest was being compromised and would never lead to the sense of freedom and restoration I'd been seeking.

I could not have been more wrong.

YOUR ESCAPE FROM INFLAMMATION

A great benefit of the *going without* aspect of all types of fasting is that it gives your body a chance to rest and do a thorough cleanup at the cellular level. Biological mechanisms that are typically occupied with digestion (including the digestion of things you would have been better off not eating in the first place) switch into self-care mode. Dead cells and tissue, fatty deposits, tumors, and other obstructions to optimal bodily function are all burned as fuel or bundled up and eliminated as waste.

A great benefit of all that cleanup, meanwhile, is that it soothes one of the most insidious and destructive processes in your body: inflammation.

Everyone has experienced inflammation, but scientists are still puzzling out exactly how it works at the cellular level. Fundamentally, inflammation is a by-product of the immune system activating itself in response to an injury or perceived threat. If you twist your ankle, for example, it turns red and becomes swollen and hot to the touch as a result of an inflammatory response intended to begin the repair and healing processes. What's happening is that your body is enlarging the tissues around the damaged area and flooding it with immune cells and proteins designed to fight disease, promote clotting, and knit together damaged tissue. That package of responses is known as *acute inflammation*, and it is the good kind.

Acute inflammation comes to the rescue quickly to destroy invading microbes, remove dead cells, and repair cellular damage. It lasts just hours or days before returning the body to a state of balance. In the first century CE, the Roman physician Aulus Celsus wrote one of the first medical encyclopedias, *De Medicina*,[1] in which he defined acute inflammation by its telltale symptoms: *dolor, rubor, functio, laesa, tumor,* and *calor.* In modern terminology, that corresponds to pain, redness, immobility, swelling, and heat, or PRISH, which is a shorthand still used to train physicians and which perfectly describes the symptoms of a sprained ankle. We would not survive long without acute inflammation; it heals wounds, builds muscle, and fights off infection.

But there is another, more disconcerting type of inflammation—the kind that can be triggered by the things we eat. Along with the essential energy needed to run our muscles and brain, many foods contain damaging molecules that stress your cells in ways similar to a physical injury, which is why they provoke a similar inflammatory response. In this case, however, there is no specific injury to heal, and the inflammation lasts as long as those damaging molecules are around. If you don't change your diet, they can stay with you for months, years, or your whole lifetime. The result is *chronic inflammation*. It is your body's self-repair system gone haywire.

On an intuitive level, it's easy to know that certain foods make us feel good and others make us feel bad. Two millennia ago, the ancient Greeks interpreted these feelings in a spiritual way: they believed that eating and drinking allowed demonic spirits into the body and embraced fasting as a way to achieve purification by keeping the demons at bay. As naive as that might sound in the modern age, they were onto something. When we eat and drink, harmful agents do enter the body. Today we call them *toxins*. If they trigger inflammation, they are referred to as inflammogens.

Chronic inflammation locks your body in a perpetual state of molecular stress as it struggles mightily to heal injuries that cannot be healed. Things go downhill from there as the inflammation response feeds on itself. Your intestinal lining becomes irritated, allowing bacteria and bits of undigested food to enter the bloodstream. The immune system correctly perceives these intruders as a problem and instigates even more of an inflammatory response. Toxins in the gut provoke the release of cell-signaling proteins known as cytokines, which are able to enter the brain and cause inflammation there as well. Adding insult to injury, a low-quality diet disrupts the Krebs cycle, the essential chain of chemical reactions that generates energy from the carbohydrates, fats, and proteins in your cells. Toxic substances interfere with the Krebs cycle, allowing electrons to leak away. Your body loses precious energy; the stray electrons, meanwhile, give rise to irritating, electrically charged molecules known as free radicals, which are another significant trigger of inflammation.

As bad as that all sounds, the medical reality of it is even worse. During chronic inflammation, the immune system floods the surrounding tissue with specialized types of white blood cells—lymphocytes, monocytes, and macrophages—to clean up the accumulating damage. Over time, these cells often end up attacking healthy tissue and organs, leading to autoimmune disease. Inflammation has been identified as an underlying factor in cancer, rheumatoid arthritis, heart disease, diabetes, Alzheimer's, and asthma. It contributes to obesity, fatty liver, and chronic kidney disease. Chronic inflammation turns your thinking foggy, and it accelerates the aging process.

But you'd never consume anything that would do those terrible things to you, right? Bad news: you probably do it all the time.

Supermarkets and convenience stores (and many restaurants as well) are crammed with foods made using low-quality, inflammation-stoking fats, such as those in corn and canola oil. Why? Because they are cheap. Big Food inexorably delivers the most easily marketable products—ones that are inexpensive, tasty, and pretty. Over the years, the industry systematically phased out expensive, high-value fats such as grass-fed butter, coconut oil, ghee, and even lard from healthy animals (lard was a part of the human diet for ages, yet until recently heart disease was rare). Your long-term health is not a part of the business plan. It takes about two years for the fats you eat to be incorporated into half of the cell membranes in your body. By then you're not going to have any idea why you don't have the energy and mental clarity you used to. Big Food won't have any idea, either.

Steering clear of all the processed foods made with those oils is really tough. Start reading some ingredient labels, and you'll see what I mean. And that's still only part of the inflammation challenge you face. You might decide that you're going to eat healthy by avoiding or minimizing obviously toxic foods such as high-fructose corn syrup, sugar, and trans fats, all of which cause inflammation. But keeping the chemical demons at bay is not that simple. Plant-based foods such as bread, and even some vegetables such as bell peppers and kale, can cause inflammation, too.

Inflammatory Foods That Cause Cravings and Make Fasting Harder

- High-oxalate foods (which can induce your body to produce calcium crystals that are hard to eliminate): sesame, soy, raw kale, spinach, chard, beets

- High-histamine foods (containing a neurotransmitter that can cause allergies and cravings): fish sauce, soy sauce, leftover fish, leftover pork

- Phytic acid (which inhibits protein digestion): beans, grains, wheat, legumes

- Burned or charred meat, grains, or vegetables: high-temperature cooking creates toxic compounds, including AGE (advanced glycation end products), HCA (heterocyclic amines), and PAH (polycyclic aromatic hydrocarbons, found in soot)[2]

- High-lectin foods allowed (not recommended but sometimes allowed) on the Bulletproof Diet: tomatoes, potatoes, bell peppers, hot peppers, eggplant, beans, chickpeas

Contrary to a common assumption, most inflammatory by-products are made by plants or microbes, not animals, for reasons that are rooted deep in the nature of evolution. If you are an animal and you don't want to be eaten, you can generally run and hide. If you are a plant, you need to defend yourself in place: you can grow a hard, protective shell, like a walnut; you can sprout spines, like a cactus; or you can fill yourself with poison. The poison strategy is a really common one. Think for a second what would happen if you were to go into your backyard or your local park, pick the first leaf you saw, and eat it. Seriously, *don't do it*! You'd very likely end up doubled over in pain.

The plant world is full of inflammatory toxins that can find their way into your food. That's true even of crop plants such as tomatoes or pumpkins, and it doesn't take much of those plants' leaves to mess you up. Back when my daughter was two years old, she ate two leaves from a pumpkin plant in our yard. She then spent the rest of the day farting and crying from cramps. Her body was reacting to proteins called lectins, which are present in many plant leaves to keep insects and predators and herbivores away. Lectin is sometimes called an antinutrient because of its harsh, inflammation-triggering effects.

The plants that contain the most toxins are the least desirable and hence the cheapest—which means they are right at the top of Big Food's shopping list. As long as it's possible to make those plants taste good and delay the bad effects so that they don't have any immediately obvious negative effects on your health, they will find their way into junk food. These days, you will find even low-quality plants being marketed as health foods. Take hummus as an example. It is full of lectins (chickpeas), but it's a cheap source of calories compared to guacamole, so you find it everywhere, even though everyone knows that guacamole is healthier (and tastes better).

A lot of people willingly—eagerly!—unleash other sources of inflammation into their bodies all of the time. You've almost certainly exposed yourself to this widespread food toxin: alcohol. Think about how you felt during a hangover. Was it painful? Were you immobilized? You can look at a hangover as inflammation in response to a common inflammatory microbial toxin from yeast. Even if you limit your drinking and build your diet around foods that don't contain inflammatory products, you may still be causing your body damage through undisciplined eating habits. Your body can become inflamed simply if you eat at the wrong time or eat too much. Both the size of your meals and their timing are very important in determining the impact of the food you eat.

This all sounds rather daunting, I realize. How can you possibly succeed when you have all of this biology and evolution and industry working against you? It's true, inflammation will kick your ass if you let it. But you have a secret weapon, one that gives you a break from toxins and inflammation across the board. Fasting kicks *inflamma-*

tion's ass, giving the digestive organs a chance to rest and reset while nothing inflammatory comes in, in the same way that we allow our muscles to recover after a hard workout.

When you fast, your body takes energy that would normally be used to digest food and redirects it to healing and repair. Your cells need nourishment and oxygen to thrive, but lifestyle choices such as being sedentary or dietary choices such as overeating or eating toxin-laden foods that result in digestive issues promote cellular degeneration and what biologists delicately call *apoptosis*. Let's just call it what it is: cell death.

A low-quality diet and inactive lifestyle will slowly kill your cells—and you. Fasting gives new life to your body. When you start fasting, one of the primary reasons that you feel better is that you've stopped consuming antinutrients. You've stopped eating bad oils. You've stopped eating the inflammogens that Big Food puts in there.

You'll start to wonder why you have so much more energy and mental clarity. Is it because of the ketones that turned down inflammation? Yes. Was it because when you stopped eating crap, it turned down inflammation? Yes. Was the power of those two together doubly powerful? Yes. Could you achieve this result even by eating a high-fat diet without any toxins in it? Yes again! I've been doing this type of diet for more than ten years, and I've taught hundreds of thousands of people how to do it successfully.

Fasting can be flexible. Avoiding inflammatory foods can be easy and enjoyable. The key is learning which foods to cut out of your diet—the ones that I call kryptonite. Whether Mother Nature made it or a chemistry lab made it, you've got to avoid kryptonite. I'm here to help you do that. You can find a more detailed list—the Bulletproof Fasting Roadmap—for free online at daveasprey.com/fastingroadmap.[3] I recommend printing it out and putting it on your fridge. In the meantime, here's the short list of kryptonite foods:

- Soy milk, fruit juice, diet drinks, soda, sports drinks

- Corn, soy, beets, chard, collards, kale, spinach, eggplant, peppers, tomatoes

- Margarine, GMO oils, industrial lard, vegetable oil, seed oil, canola oil, peanut oil, cottonseed oil, sunflower oil, safflower oil

- Powdered milk, evaporated milk, soy protein, wheat protein

- Packaged salad dressings and sauces, caseinate, hydrolyzed gluten, MSG, hydrolyzed yeast

To be clear, you can eat all these things and still benefit from fasting. It's just a lot harder because you'll be hungry all the time. Once you are liberated from kryptonite, you can become superhuman. During the biochemical cleansing process, your intestines, vital organs, and even your bloodstream will be purified. Diseased cells will be replaced by healthy tissue. This doesn't just make you feel better, it might actually make you *look* better. All that new, healthy tissue can give you a more youthful appearance.

DAVID AND HIS FOOD GOLIATH

At this point, I'd like to share a little bit more about my journey to wellness, because a lot of it involved my own battle with inflammation and a wonky metabolism. Frankly, when I started out, my health was a shit show (that's the scientific term for it). But if I could fix my body, you can, too. In fact, your path is probably going to be a lot easier than mine.

When I was five years old, my family moved from California to New Mexico. We had no idea that the walls inside our new home were filled with toxic mold or that the abandoned gold and silver mines in the nearby desert where I liked to shoot guns (this was back before video games) were loaded with heavy-metal toxins, including lead and mercury. All I knew was that things were starting to go wrong with me. By the time I was fourteen, my body was breaking down so badly that I had chronic arthritis in both knees, persistent nosebleeds, and recurring bouts of strep throat. By my early twenties I was obese, squeezing into an XXL T-shirt, and even a triple pleat on my pants couldn't hide the fat. I tried a bunch of diets. I worked out for ninety minutes every day for eighteen months straight, but I still couldn't lose weight. The symptoms that scared me most were crippling fatigue and brain fog—I was always exhausted and had a hard time focusing on my career.

In my late twenties, my doctor ran lab tests and told me that I was prediabetic and at high risk for a stroke and heart attack. In addition, I had hypothyroidism; this is a type of autoimmune disease in which my immune system was attacking my thyroid gland, so it wasn't producing enough thyroid hormone. My dysfunctional thyroid led to a slow metabolic rate, the symptoms of which included being tired and putting on weight very easily. Although I was not yet thirty, I had a body more like that of a declining sixty-year-old.

The root cause of this pain, lethargy, and obesity was inflammation. I got hit especially early and hard by it, but inflammation affects all of us to some degree and more as we age. If you pay attention each morning, you'll notice that the size of your belly sometimes grows overnight—that's inflammation. The same type of swelling happens in your brain; you just can't see it. These changes are caused by cell-signaling molecules called cytokines. Researchers discovered them in the 1950s, but only within the past couple decades have they began to understand the link between inflammation and cytokines—specifically, a group of them called (of course) inflammatory cytokines,[4] which are present throughout the body.

While all that was going on inside of me, I just wanted to live a normal life. I was worn out by my endless diseases and by the emotional baggage that comes with having so many health problems. But it was becoming increasingly obvious that if I didn't do something to change the trajectory of my health, things weren't going to end well; the time had come to take action. My first step was admitting that all of the solutions that were supposed to help me lose weight (such as low-fat diets and chronic cardio exercise) weren't doing anything for me.

I spent four years immersed in research. The first place it led me was to the Atkins diet, more generally known as a ketogenic diet, which emphasizes cutting sugar and carbs while consuming protein and fat in order to get the body into a state of ketosis. It's the grand-father of the modern keto diet, which still suffers from many of the limitations of the Atkins diet. That's because it doesn't fully address the issue of inflammation. But it got me started on a better path. I lost 50 pounds in the first three months of what would now be labeled a "dirty keto" diet. It was like a miracle.

Losing the other 50 pounds took me ten years. Why? Because those first 50 pounds were fat, but dieting to eliminate the fat didn't address the much more intractable problem of inflammation. Without knowing it, I was eating ketogenic foods that were also inflammatory. Nobody told me about kryptonite. Learning how to get rid of inflam-mation through fasting was a whole other journey for me. (News flash: when you're eating *nothing*, you're also eating *nothing inflammatory*.)

Even now, a bunch of the modern keto evangelists cling to the same flawed philosophy of the Atkins diet. The dirty keto diet allows, or even encourages, eating highly processed, highly packaged foods just to stay in ketosis. Anything that's not a carb is keto, which means that wheat gluten (which is protein) qualifies as keto on this diet. Vegetable oil is keto, too. Technically speaking, that's absolutely true. The problem is, wheat gluten and vegetable oil make you fat. Gluten also causes inflammation, and there's some evidence that vegetable oil can, too. Both of them make you hungry. Seed oils definitely cause inflammation, as I noted earlier. There's a common perception that eating any kind of fat for fuel on the ketogenic diet is healthy, but if the fat you're consuming is inflammatory, you defeat the purpose.

Fasting provides an easy framework for not only when to eat but also what to eat. You can have your morning coffee with MCT oil and butter. You will *not* be eating gluten and vegetable oil and pro-cessed foods. You *will* be giving your body a break from inflammation and all of its associated health problems. Heart disease is actually more strongly associated with inflammation than with cholesterol level. Coronary disease accounts for an estimated 31 percent of global mortality, according to the World Health Organization[5]—and long periods of time without food have been shown to reduce the risk of developing it by lowering blood pressure and triglycerides in addition to inflammation.

This point bears repeating: fasting reduces inflammation, improves health, and boosts your self-control *no matter what kind of eating regimen you prefer.* It will help you out if you're on dirty keto, if you're vegan, or if you're living on a pizza and nachos diet. Still, I'd prefer that you eat clean if you're going to stay in ketosis. You'll see better results, reduce inflammation as much as possible, and you'll just feel better.

How can you tell if your body is inflamed? The short answer is: if you're eating a typical modern diet full of processed foods, you're inflamed on some level. The most dangerous forms of inflammation—such as an inflamed brain, heart, or liver—can be hard to detect with the naked eye, but some inflammation is visible right on the surface. Take a look in the mirror. Do your love handles change from day to day? That's inflammation. Is your skin puffy or full of acne? That's inflammation. Is your grip weak, or are your joints or back sore when you wake up? That's inflammation, too.

After I lost the weight, I needed to find a way to keep it off. That meant I had to win the battle against inflammatory foods. The problem was, I didn't know which foods were making me inflamed, and back then there was limited research available to guide me. Despite my best efforts, I was still suffering from inflammation. I could see it in the puffiness of my muffin top. I could feel it when I woke up with aching joints that made it painful to walk.

I dialed in on the causes of inflammation. I took a good hard look at every single thing I ate and researched how it affected my body. I did day-to-day comparison tests on myself when necessary. I learned how to turn off my hunger by *not* eating certain foods, and that knowledge was the basis of *The Bulletproof Diet.* And along the way I discovered intermittent fasting.

Well, no one alive today actually *discovered* intermittent fasting; it's been a part of our species for as long as we have been a species. It's just that I discovered how it worked for me, and I did discover that using coffee with butter and MCT oil produced extremely powerful results, better than fasting alone when I started out. I'm pretty sure no one else alive or dead had hit upon that weird combination!

When I began intermittent fasting, it was like turning on a light switch. Back then, there were no blogs about it and no books. I knew that the Atkins diet recommended a "fat fast" to get into ketosis, but it was cheese based and used artificial sweeteners, so I hacked it. I already knew that Bulletproof Coffee made me feel great, so I had it for breakfast to kick off ketosis. Just by skipping breakfast and making my morning coffee Bulletproof, I lost more weight and didn't even want lunch. When I skipped breakfast and had no Bulletproof Coffee, on the other hand, I got distractingly hungry at 11:30 in the morning and didn't function well at work. It's such a simple behavioral change, one that everybody is capable of doing: just go sixteen hours without eating anything inflammatory at all. Almost like magic, the anti-inflammation systems in the body start to kick in right away. (Except that it's not magic at all; this is exactly how your body has evolved to work if you will just let it.) You get a rest from inflammatory food toxins. At the same time, your body switches into ketosis and you get a metabolic reconditioning.

For you, going on a basic sixteen-hour fast may well be the first time you've ever experienced a taste of life without new inflammation. Like me, you will probably become aware that you have food addictions. These are not just emotional attachments; they are true biological addictions to certain molecules and foods. Make no mistake: these addictions will be hard to break. If you have a biological addiction, milk protein can be as hard to quit as nicotine. Your body will fight back when you try to quit. The Big Food industry will make sure you see ads for those foods everywhere and that they are easy to grab when you go into the supermarket or drugstore. As soon as you start fasting, though, you start to assert control over them.

Two of the most common biological addictions are to wheat (gluten) and dairy products. You may think you don't have to worry about them because you're not allergic to either one. Truth is, you probably have no idea what effect they're having on you. How many times have you gone three days without eating wheat or dairy protein? (Butter contains a negligible amount of protein.) Both gluten and dairy products have known inflammatory effects. You'll never learn the impact they have on your body until you break your addictions, which is a lot harder than it sounds.

The gluten proteins in bread and the casein proteins in milk and cheese often break down in the body into molecules known as gluteo-morphin and casomorphin. Notice the "morphin" part of their names? These molecules are both morphine analogs that trigger the opioid receptors in your brain—your brain's pleasure centers. In other words, the way your body processes the high of eating a grilled cheese sandwich is a lot like the way it does a shot of heroin. The two produce different levels of euphoria, obviously, but both deliver an addictive sensation of gratification. That's why when you eat bread, you're going to want bread the next day and the next day and the next day. That's why it's so easy to fill up on the breadbasket at the beginning of a meal in a restaurant. Your body craves that opiate sensation. Try fasting while thinking about crusty French bread.

If you've trained your body for years that every morning it will get its fix—buttered toast, maybe, or a muffin, or milk poured over cereal made of grain—you're probably going to get a little bit twitchy when you start intermittent fasting and deprive the body of that fix. That's fine. It's a manageable craving.

When your body starts asking "Where's my hit of gluten?" you can respond, "Hey buddy, I'm giving you the gift of sixteen hours to repair yourself. It's time for spring cleaning. You've got nothing else to do, so you might as well turn all the energy you were using to combat the inflammation from the food I was giving you into more enzyme production. Let's perform a systems upgrade."

THE JOYOUS EXPERIMENT

Around the time I was learning about the tremendous impact of inflammation and had begun to experiment with fasting, I went on a spiritual retreat in a remote region of western Tibet. During the trip, I'd been fasting and eating almost nothing bad for me—not out of choice, so much, but because there was very little food available at all. Halfway along the sacred path around Mount Kailash, I was offered yak butter tea, which is given to travelers to help prevent altitude sickness (I was 18,000 feet above sea level). To my amazement, I felt great afterward. I later found out that blending butter into the tea can do powerful things for inflammation and energy production.

It turns out that taking a brief period away from food does not lead to a sense of "I'm going to die." What I was actually thinking up there on Mount Kailash was "Wow, this is what it's like to have limitless energy and feel great." That's one of the most surprising, immediate benefits of reducing your inflammation.

Activating the power of fasting is not that simple, however. If it were, everybody would be doing intermittent fasts already. If you do a prolonged fast, especially a "dry" fast with no water or other liquids, the elation passes. Even a short fast can be seriously unpleasant if you jump into it unprepared. It starts to seem as though your fears about fasting are coming true. Your superpowers are replaced with nagging voices of hunger, fatigue, and irritability. The question becomes "How can these things be managed?" and then "*Can* they be managed?"

The answer eluded me for quite some time. I couldn't figure out how to re-create the surge of energy that ran through my body on Mount Kailash. I had watched how Tibetan people could subsist on little more than a few cups of yak butter tea each day, yet carry more than I could through freezing temperatures for twelve hours without more food. They weren't strictly fasting, but it was close. I researched different styles of fasting and introduced a regular discipline of fasting into my life. I tried fasting for four days, twenty-four-hour fasting, fasting with and without coffee, tea, and butter. And on and on, until I discovered the biohacks that work to create more energy than I know what to do with.

Part one of the answer is Bulletproof Coffee, a concoction inspired by the yak butter tea I drank in Tibet. This is the difference between a Bulletproof Fast and a regular fast. It allows you to experience more of the inflammation-free euphoria and near-zero hunger, and it minimizes the energy dip most people encounter when going without food.

Part two is embracing that idea that fasting is not just one thing; there are many styles of fasting and many rhythms of intermittent fasting. All of them provide anti-inflammatory and other benefits. If your fast allows some flexibility, it's a lot more likely to fit in with the rest of your life. In my case, I have kids, and I'm the CEO of a good-sized company. Planning a forty-eight-hour fast isn't always easy. Sometimes it works best when the kids and my wife go skiing or do something else that I don't. (I have screws in my knee; that's a whole other story.) Or I'll do the same thing sometimes on business trips. Afterward, I always feel better and get that feeling of rejuvenation. The difference is the lack of inflammation.

Part three is drawing on your social support network, especially when you first start doing intermittent fasting. You can easily find apps and online communities to help you out, but I really recommend that you find a buddy who wants to try fasting with you. Social bonding is yet another way to reduce inflammation, by the way. In 2020, a group of researchers at the University of Surrey and at Brunel University London found that social isolation is associated with increased inflammation in the body. Isolated people showed elevated levels of C-reactive protein, a protein produced in the liver, which normally floods tissues after an injury. It also elevates levels of fibrinogen, which promotes blood clotting. The research team also found that the link between social isolation and inflammation was stronger among men than women.[6] You'll read more about the gender differences in fasting in chapter 9.

Part four drives home the point I made earlier: don't look at fasting as a burdensome chore to lose weight or to tend to your health. You will probably lose weight, and you definitely will be healthier—but neither of those things will happen if the fast makes you so miserable that you quit. That's why friends, flexibility, and a well-timed Bulletproof Coffee are so essential. They let you experience what it is to be freed from the demon of inflammation. You *get to* fast, you don't *have to*.

If fasting brings pleasure instead of misery, you'll keep doing it—not because you swore an oath you'd keep going, but because you'll want to keep feeling good. And once you feel good more of the time, you'll be more likely to make other changes that reduce inflammation and enhance your sense of well-being: making better food choices, exercising regularly, avoiding smoking, reducing or quitting alcohol consumption, and getting enough sleep. Taking short breaks from food is part of a broader program of steering yourself away from self-destructive tendencies.

Look at fasting, then, as a decision to be in charge of yourself and work toward being your best self. Fasting makes your body work better. It makes you tougher. It makes you more resilient. It prepares you mentally to take on everything in the world. We all say we want to live a long life, right? But what we all really want is an enduring *high-quality life*. Fasting is central to both parts: living long and living well.

For decades, many leading biologists promoted the idea that human longevity is largely controlled by our genes. If your parents and their parents and their parents before them all lived into their nineties, for instance, there was a good chance you would, too. Your family had "good genes," whatever those might be. On the other hand, if your ancestors didn't make it past their fifties, well, too bad for you. Several major research groups continue to sequence the genomes of centenarians, searching for quirks in their DNA that could account for their extreme longevity. Researchers working on the New England Centenarian Study have flagged more than a hundred genetic variants that preferentially show up among the oldest old.[7]

But mostly what such studies have revealed is that genes are just a single, somewhat ambiguous component in the mix of factors that determine health and longevity. Diet, lifestyle, and other daily choices are just as important—and not necessarily in the ways you might think. Mikhail Blagosklonny, a gerontologist at the Roswell Park Cancer Institute in Buffalo, New York, is a leading proponent of the once-controversial theory that certain types of weak stresses, including fasting, can extend life span by activating the body's self-repair mechanisms. "Life span can be extended by either (a) slowing down aging [or] (b) by increasing aging tolerance," he declared in one influential paper.[8] In his view and the view of a growing number of his colleagues, increasing aging tolerance is exactly what weak stresses do.

Experiment after experiment has demonstrated that animals tend to live longer when underfed, whereas if they are given all the food they want to survive, they have demonstrably shorter life spans. In the laboratory setting, this underfeeding technique is known as *caloric restriction*. It's an extreme version of the insidious "calories in, calories out," or CICO, diets that have recently developed an unfortunate following. It typically involves giving the animals about 30 percent fewer calories than in their baseline diet. What the science doesn't tell you is which calories to cut or how to cut them. Some antiaging obsessives have tried to apply the lab techniques to human diets, simply cutting calories across the board. It's similar in approach to some of the old-fashioned calorie-counting diets, which told people that the way to lose weight and stay thin was to remain hungry—pretty much forever.

No wonder people almost never stayed on those diets for long. Just as CICO diets are the very definition of misery, so, too, are long-term caloric-restricted diets, especially if you ignore what food makes up the calories you're eating. It might be worth it if it was the only way to live a lot longer, at least for some people. But for most of us, calorie restriction and the suffering that comes with it just aren't tolerable over time. That's why intermittent fasting is so exciting. When you do a smart intermittent fast, you're probably going to end up eating less overall—not because you're forcing yourself but because you're just not as hungry as you used to be. In the early days after I developed the Bulletproof Diet, many people thought it worked just because people were eating less. Now we can show what's actually happening; there are hormonal changes and inflammation changes associated with the fasting process and with the diet itself. But you often do end up reducing your calorie intake as well, and you get the knock-on benefits of that, too. You may end up cutting close to the number of calories that people on calorie-restricted diets do—you just do it with more energy and joy and better health as a bonus. It boils down to a simple formula: Eat good-quality food until you're full. Stop for a while. Do it again. Enjoy a better quality of life.

And you probably will have more of that life. You know how your brain feels exhausted at the end of a long, busy day? Well, it genuinely is exhausted at the cellular level. The nonstop firing of your neurons creates waste products that have to be disposed of. A fast of at least twelve (ideally eighteen) hours gives your cells the signal that it's time to clean house. Likewise, your mitochondria need regular periods of rest, repair, and regeneration. The textbook description that the mitochondria are the "powerhouses of the cells" is a cliché, but it's true: these little capsule-shaped structures are found inside almost all of the cells in your body, and they generate most of the chemical energy in your body, storing it in a molecule called adenosine triphosphate, or ATP. The mitochondria are the prime movers behind your metabolism. You need well-fueled, plentiful mitochondria in order to stay energized, mentally focused, and happy.

Reduced function of the mitochondria is connected to the symptoms of aging we most dread, including fatigue, increased body fat, and declining cognitive ability. Researchers have found links between mitochondrial dysfunction and nearly every age-related disease, including Alzheimer's and cardiovascular disease. Tying all of these strands together, a recent study led by medical researchers at Cambridge University showed that mitochondria act as tiny switches that toggle the inflammation response in the body.[9] Healthy mitochondria do a better job regulating your inflammatory and anti-inflammatory systems. When they're in good working order, all of your other biological systems do a better job of taking care of you, too.

The bottom line is that fasting reduces inflammation, promotes regeneration, and makes you feel younger and more energetic. Fasting makes you harder to kill. More important, it gives you more to live for.

TRUTH TIME: WHY YOU SHOULD FAST

It is truly remarkable how fasting can troubleshoot your biology, boost your energy, and cut your risk of disease. I want you to have all of these benefits. But I'm also a realist who has guided a lot of people into intermittent fasting and watched some of them fail to stick with it. The only way you'll cut inflammation and tighten up your Krebs cycle is if you find a way to make fasting satisfying for you—not at a molecular level but at a personal level. It's not about the science. It's about *you*, and you're more than science.

People almost always claim that they care about their health. But if someone hands you a bagel—or shows you a picture of a sexy person or shows you a way to make a ton of money—the concept of health will probably fly right out of your mind as those new motivations jump to the top of your priority list. Cravings are extremely effective at making us forget our goals and our priorities. Even if you are trying to take good care of yourself, it's really hard to remain mindful of your health all of the time. Otherwise, tending to your health is probably around number seven on your "honey-do" list.

Instead of fighting against reality, let's try some radical honesty: You are not going to fast just for your health. And you're certainly not going to fast if it makes you miserable. You shouldn't even try to make *health* your guiding motivation. That may sound strange, given the messages you hear all the time in books and articles and on TV shows. It's a nonstop drumbeat: "You've got to do this exercise or eat this superfood or follow this complicated diet so that you can be healthier. You must, if you want to take care of yourself! If you don't, that must mean you don't care about yourself!"

None of it is true. None of it lines up with the way the mind and body really work. Your desire for great health is not as biologically strong as your need for safety, satisfaction, connection with other people, or even power and success. No judgments here. I'm describing deep-seated human psychology that we all share: you, me, everyone you know.

Take the social aspects of food, for example. People like to go out to eat because they need to connect with other people. That's a powerful motivation. Sure, you might master the self-control to remind yourself that you're fasting for your health, and that reminder might enable you to maintain your fast during a social occasion—but damn, it's hard to say no when someone passes you a plate of fried whatever. Giving in doesn't make you weak or a bad person. Food is one key method through which human beings connect. Denying yourself human connection is a really bad use of your power of self-control.

That need to connect reminds me of the days when so many people decided that they would get healthy by running a marathon. Many of the newly enlisted runners were heavily overweight and not conditioned. Their outrageous scheme was to go from being total nonathletes, unable to do so much as jog around the block, to running the 26.2 miles of a full marathon. They convinced their friends to join them in order to experience camaraderie. Then they all started training. Amazingly, a lot of them managed to complete their goal and run an entire marathon—just not for the reason they thought. Mostly, they believed that they were running for their health. In reality, they were running to satisfy their deep desire for connection.

If you've ever made it to the finish line of an endurance event like that, you probably know that a sudden decision to run a marathon is really rough on you. Simply running the 26.2 miles doesn't work very well as a health and wellness plan. Look at the bulk of the runners who are doing it. They may accomplish the challenge, but if you pay attention to the many body types in a pack of first-time marathoners, you'll see a whole lot of metabolic issues that are not fixed by running a marathon.

To be sure, you'll probably feel better about yourself if you complete a huge physical challenge such as a marathon. You will get a boost in confidence just by proving that you can go the distance. We often feel compelled to enter such extreme events to show ourselves that we're in charge of our own biology, that we can to do anything. But keep in mind that 80 percent of people who take up long-distance running experience a significant injury in the first year. Heck, the ancient Greek guy who ran the first marathon died after 26.2 miles of running—not exactly a recipe for health. I'm not saying that long-distance running won't work for you—it might—but oftentimes we enter one of these events for the wrong reasons. We approach them as a symbol of achievement rather than as part of a consistent set of decisions for creating and maintaining a healthy lifestyle.

There's a better way to put yourself in charge.

If you want to feel better about yourself and gain the ability to control your willpower (I'm not going to call it "empowerment," because it implies that someone else has to give you the power), fasting is the key. You can start small. First, go a morning without food. Then, when you've mastered that, go a day without food. I promise you that you'll feel a distinct sensation of achievement. Just like a runner upping his or her mileage to run a marathon, you can then move up to some of the more advanced fasting techniques. You may think you can't, but you can. Each time you successfully complete a fast, you'll discover that it isn't even that hard and the results are worth it. You'll feel a sense of achievement and success. Your clothes will fit better, too.

Fasting is also a lot healthier for you than running a marathon. Or a triathlon, or whatever your big race might be. *Fasting is better for you both psychologically and physically.* Rather than getting a bunch of friends together for a run around your local park, ask the same people to join you in your fast. The only reason that sentence looks weird is that it is probably the first time anybody has ever suggested this idea to you. Fasting together is more important than doing endurance exercise together, but you can do both.

There's something truly beautiful about connecting with a couple friends and saying, "Hey, let's do this thing together." The kind of fasting I'm talking about leaves room for social interactions. You can still meet up for "breakfast"—but skip the pancakes and instead grab a coffee (and you can treat yourself to really good coffee, since you're saving money on food!). Instead of a boozy happy hour after work, soaking up inflammatory alcohol, you can meet up with your friends for a workout or a game of softball or Frisbee—something that actually makes your body feel good and is a better bonding activity than pounding beers and nachos.

This way, instead of feeling deprived of social engagement, you rewrite the rules of social engagement to work for you. You're making a new kind of human connection. And when you cross the finish line and complete your fast together, the sense of achievement will be huge and totally counterintuitive. You won't feel hungry and cranky like people on calorie-restriction diets. Instead, you'll feel your physical and mental best. Above all, your body will be a lot less inflamed, which means that the things that always hurt will stop hurting. There's a good chance you'll discover pains you never knew you had; you'll notice their absence because suddenly you'll feel so much better.

Notice that none of this requires fixating on your health. Ultimately, your job is to be a high-performance human being so that you can enjoy all of the things that make your life meaningful. Doing that job right requires changing your connection with food so that you can tame inflammation and the other processes in your body that are currently holding you back. You have to learn new tricks that will let you master your cravings in ways that make you feel better than you did before.

An important part of that mastery will be getting used to spending time with people while they eat but you don't. You'll soon realize three things: First, you can still laugh and tell stories and enjoy relationships with other people even if there's no food on your plate. Second, we don't all need to refuel our bodies at the same time! If you don't care that you're not eating, chances are your friends won't care, either. Third, some people will feel as though *they're* starving when they see you fasting, and they'll stop at nothing to try to feed you. My only advice here is to simply stick with your plan and respond to skeptics with honesty and love.

Sitting down to a meal with friends and family is a fundamentally meaningful ritual, and I would never suggest you stop doing it. Eating with other people when your body doesn't want or won't benefit from the food on the table isn't a great experience, so when you do have a communal meal, enjoy it. Just don't obligate yourself to eat in ways that you know are toxic for your body.

Break that pattern. Don't break the fast. Take all the gifts that come with fasting—less bloated inflammation, more energy and confidence—and focus on the things that will make you feel your best.

3

MANY STAGES AND MANY STYLES OF FASTING

When you're embarking on a spiritual journey, sometimes you need to let go and allow things to happen however they're going to. You have to leave room for serendipity. Delilah put that serendipity principle to the test when she told me I'd be doing my solitary (solitary!) vision quest in the same cave as another seeker. It would be fine, the shaman assured me, as long as we both followed the rules. Rule number one: the two of us were not allowed to talk to each other in the cave. Well, yeah.

I went along with her plan, though all the while I was wondering how I was going to attain the transcendence that I had come for. The idea of experiencing true solitude while there was another person in the cave seemed as improbable to me as the idea of being able to eat while fasting. In that spirit, I almost stuffed a protein bar into my backpack ("just in case, for emergencies," I told myself) before we headed out. It was only at the last minute that I left it behind at the shaman's house: a wave of self-control came over me, and I removed the temptation so I could follow through on my full intent. Plus, the year was 2008, and protein bars tasted like crap back then.

Delilah drove us to the cave in her beat-up old pickup truck, looking a bit like a movie cowboy in her overalls—complete with a weathered tan and cowboy hat—and dropped us off. Before departing, she reminded my partner and me to keep space from each other, long before social distancing was a thing, and also to keep our phones powered off. The sole exception to the no-phones rule was that we were expected to power up for precisely one minute each morning in order to receive a text message from her and let her know we were okay. Thankfully, smartphones did not exist yet, so there were no other ways we could distract ourselves while we were in the cave. Except by talking. Or making hand signals.

The shaman also intoned somewhat mysteriously that she would be "checking in on us remotely," whatever that meant. When I asked her what she was talking about, she gave a little smile and told me, "I will know how you're doing." Despite my attempts to pry more of an explanation out of her, she refused to say anything else. I didn't find any hidden cameras in the cave, though.

Walking into the cave took me into a most cosmic aspect of the fasting world—the initial inspiration behind the book you are reading now.

PAY NO MIND TO THE CALORIE COPS

In the personal quest for strength and wellness, people often confuse fasting and dieting. The two certainly overlap in the general sense: Both involve *going without*, and in both cases you will probably lose weight and maybe consume fewer calories, too. But fundamentally, they are vastly different—as different as going into a cave alone and going into a cave with someone else. Fasting directly addresses the cravings that are holding you back. Dieting has the power to make them even worse.

The pervasive culture of dieting is a major impediment that holds people back from fasting or leads them to do it in unproductive ways. It is one reason I struggled so mightily with my weight in my twenties, losing weight only to put it right back on again. I was already feeling bad, both physically and psychologically, and dieting didn't help matters. Nothing makes you feel more like a failure than enduring suffering to lose 25 pounds, only to gain them back in a few weeks, plus a dozen more. The goal of diet culture is to make you feel as though a better you is just out of reach. That's one of the many reasons why the "calories in, calories out" model, commonly abbreviated as CICO, should be relegated to the dustbin of failed science. This approach treats your body as though it's a meat robot when in reality it's a dynamic system that responds to calories differently based on their source, the time they're consumed, and the unique physiological makeup of the person consuming them. Yet the myth lives on, leaving obesity, shame, and suffering in its wake.

There's also some dubious science behind CICO, much of which can be traced back to a hugely influential physiologist named Ancel Keys. In the 1930s and '40s he became obsessed with diet and starvation and tried to develop rigorous principles for proper eating. One result is that he invented the K-rations used to feed US Navy personnel during World War II (the *K* stands for "Keys"). Keys became convinced that obesity is a direct result of taking in too many calories, and he therefore advocated a low-fat, calorie-limited diet. Strangely, he did not see sugar as a problem and vigorously argued against the harmful effects of sugar when other researchers brought them to light; his arguments were finally, definitively debunked only a decade ago. Keys's ideas were greatly amplified in the 1970s, when a US Senate committee chaired by George McGovern enshrined them into a series of federal dietary recommendations and the misguided "food pyramid" that was supposed to illustrate healthy eating choices.[1]

The CICO diet and its variants grew directly out of Keys's regimented ideas about calories and obesity—including his idea that all calories are the same. Those ideas led to a clinical, unsympathetic attitude toward overweight people, which remains a central part of the ideology of the calorie counters—or, as I like to call them, the calorie police. They promote a narrative that says: If you're fat, it's because you eat too much. Because you're weak. Period. The actual data, and the actual experience that I've lived, say otherwise: if you're fat, it's because your body is not effectively turning food and air into energy; instead, it is storing fat in your tissues. (In fact, inflammation is *always* at its root a biochemical problem involving inefficiently turning air and food into electrons.) You have a metabolic problem, not a willpower problem.

If you fall for the calorie myth, you will become disheartened when the inevitable force of hunger starts to beat you down. Every time you say no to the voice in your head that tells you to eat, it will merely come back louder. And every time you muster the conviction to deny it, you're using up precious energy. You're literally using up your electrons—the chemical energy that you get from activating the Krebs cycle to digest your food—in your efforts to eat less food. Not to mention that you're spending time and focus and willpower on a losing battle when you could be allocating those resources to other important things in your life. It makes zero sense, and it's unsustainable. It's unsustainable because no one told you that eating just a little bit of most foods (and focusing on those foods obsessively) will cause a lot more hunger than eating nothing at all.

Eventually you're going to give up. You will run out of willpower, and you will run out of energy to expend on fighting. This is why almost everyone who loses weight by cutting calories gains the weight back, generally sooner rather than later. A few people do manage to succeed with a CICO strategy. They are the outliers whose stories are plastered all over the news stories and the ads—until they put the weight back on later. They manage to make calorie restriction diets work by emphasizing the rules and the process—by outsourcing their willpower and by locking their food away in cabinets. But experiments show that over the long term, people on low-calorie diets, generally speaking, are incredibly unhappy. They get depressed. They learn to fetishize their constant gnawing hunger. They tend to feel cold all the time, a starvation response in which the body lowers its core temperature to conserve energy.

The results are disconcertingly similar to those of the famous Minnesota Starvation Experiment conducted toward the end of World War II. In that study, a group of thirty-six conscientious objectors followed a drastically reduced diet designed to make them lose one quarter of their body weight. It was carried out by none other than our old friend Ancel Keys. His goal was to understand the effects of wartime starvation and recovery; the results also provided a textbook example of what extreme calorie restriction does to the body. The consequences of the diet included depression, irritability, lethargy, apathy, cold intolerance, reduced sex drive, dizziness, hair loss, tinnitus, muscle soreness, clumsiness, lack of focus, and (predictably) an endless obsession with food.[2]

Ninety-nine percent of the people reading this book would probably say, "I'd rather die than live that life." I'm one of them. There is some evidence that long-term caloric restriction can extend life span. But who wants to walk around feeling cold, sore, and foggy, distracted by a constant, gnawing hunger, while trying to convince yourself that these feelings are normal and somehow good for you?

Regardless of what they're called or how they are packaged, CICO-style diets are just not good for you, because they don't establish a healthy relationship between you and your food. Truthfully, they don't establish any relationship at all, since they reduce food to nothing more than an arbitrary number of calories. Big Food loves CICO because it provides an excuse to package crappy, inexpensive junk ingredients as health foods as long as they are low in calories. CICO diets don't train you to pay attention to what foods you eat, when you eat them, and how they affect you. They don't put you in charge of your life. Fasting works much better when you learn to eat based on hunger, not calories or cravings.

When you think about it closely, the fixation on calories and calories alone makes no sense. I promise you that 100 calories of Cheetos or 100 calories of soda do not have the same effect on your body as 100 calories of fresh coconut or, frankly, 100 calories of grass-fed beef. Here's a simple experiment to see if I'm right—I'm suggesting it here just as a thought experiment, but you could easily do it for real. Try out a CICO diet, taking in your required quantity of calories. If you're allotted 2,000 calories a day, get all of that—just do it as nothing but soda for a couple days, and see how you feel. If you still feel the same, you must be superhuman. Captain Sugar. No normal person can pass that test. Timing also matters. Try eating all of your calories at midnight for two weeks and see how much weight you gain. Then try eating the exact same number of calories at noon for two weeks. The difference will be shocking.

You don't need to know the biochemical explanations of why all calories are not created equal. You just need common sense. You have just disproven the calorie myth!

In the end, CICO-style diets don't even do the single thing they are allegedly designed to do: make you thin. The calorie police will insist, "You really can lose weight if you simply pay attention to calories in, calories out." Except that when I did that—when I genuinely went on a low-calorie, low-fat diet, complete with Entenmann's low-fat cake and all that, and I worked out an hour and a half a day, six days a week, for eighteen months—I was still fat. My triple-pleated, 46-inch-waist pants never got too big for me.

The reason CICO diets don't work is that your body has a set-point weight that is tied to ghrelin, the hunger hormone that you read about in the previous chapter, and to another molecule called CCK (cholecystokinin), which is your satiety hormone. When you have a high level of CCK in your bloodstream and a low ghrelin level, you feel good and are genuinely not hungry. If you are a 300-pound person, your ghrelin and CCK levels—that is, your body's innate hunger point—are set as though you're a 300-pound person. If you lose a bunch of weight by cutting calories, the hunger point inside you is *still* set as though you're a 300-pound person. If you starve yourself to weigh 200 pounds, you will have the gnawing hunger of a 300 pounder. That hunger will win out against your self-control. It is inevitable.

You can hold it off for a day, certainly. You can probably keep it going for ten days. You cannot hold off the hunger and all the other starvation symptoms for six months or a year. They will come creeping back relentlessly. This is exactly the wrong way to embrace *going without*. If you think that people trying to quit smoking or people trying to quit drinking have a hard time, just try to quit eating permanently! That's what your body thinks you're doing if you go on a CICO diet. You will never find your better self this way. *Small portions of most foods will make you hungrier.*

I say these things as a former fat person who is no longer fat. The reason I'm not fat anymore is that I'm not hungry anymore. It's not because I eat fewer calories! I did learn to say no to food, but in the right way—in a way that works with rather than against the biological systems inside me, by doing without food at the right time and for the right period of time. That's what intermittent fasting is. Bulletproof Intermittent Fasting in particular is designed to get your ketones up so that you'll feel much better than you would if you just blindly cut down on calories. C8 MCT oil contains calories, yet it enables you to fast longer and very likely lose weight, because it provides ketones that turn off hunger while simultaneously resetting your hunger set point to your current weight.

Here's another example of the stark difference between dieting and fasting, based on an experiment I ran on myself. Ten years ago, while I was doing research for my 2014 book *The Bulletproof Diet* (the first big book that described ketosis with intermittent fasting), I decided to test my theory that the effects of fasting are more powerful than the effects of calorie consumption. I intentionally did everything wrong from the standpoint of the calorie-counting police. I ate a staggering 4,500 calories a day and kept doing it for a month, but for breakfast I had only Bulletproof Coffee with *tons* of butter to raise the number of calories in it. I cut my sleep to less than five hours a night, which triggers obesity. I stopped exercising. But I continued my program of intermittent fasting as I did all those things.

By the straight, Ancel Keys–style accounting of the CICO diet, I should have gained about 20 pounds. I was hoping I'd gain only 3 pounds or so. That would have poked a big enough hole in CICO that I'd feel vindicated. The results were even more startling: I actually lost weight. I felt amazing. I found that I could sustain my high-calorie diet for months and months and months, to the point where I was just sick of eating. It's actually quite hard to eat 4,500 calories a day, chomping on big steaks all the time and putting extra butter on everything. After a while, I grew weary of all that eating, but I felt good. Excess calories aren't good for you even if you can handle them, however.

The experiment proved to me how powerful intermittent fasting could be, even with Bulletproof Coffee, if you apply it to your regular diet, regardless of what it is. Probably you're not eating 4,500 calories a day, but if you are, intermittent fasting will help you out. If you never wanted to restrict your calorie intake—or if you tried it and failed—fasting offers a stealth way to reduce calories as a by-product, not an end goal, of improving the way you eat. And if you are already restricting calories, intermittent fasting can give you the same benefits but in a healthier and happier way.

Here's one more crucial distinction between dieting and fasting: CICO diets force you to build your life around rigid rules; they make you accountable to the calorie-counting police; intermittent fasting encourages you to play with your methodology. It's safe to play around this way, and it's fun to do so. You are in charge of yourself.

There may come a moment when you say, "I thought I was fasting, but it didn't really work today. I got really hungry, so I gave in and ate a potato chip." When that moment comes, you will respond one of two ways. In the CICO philosophy, you would punish yourself: "Today I failed, so I will do twelve minutes of penance on the treadmill to 'pay for' those calories." That reaction doesn't do you any good. All it does is make you feel bad about yourself. Plus, there's no real way to pedal away a bag of potato chips.

In the intermittent fasting philosophy, you turn that perceived failure into a victory. Instead of telling yourself that you're a loser and wallowing in your lack of success, tell yourself that you're having a potato chip fast. You ate only one potato chip all day long—just one!—and that was the entire amount of food you ate that day. It turns out that you *can* eat just one, and you'll be *less* hungry than if you eat ten.

A lovely member of my family who looks suspiciously like my wife, Dr. Lana, was doing a five-day fast but had a teaspoon of ice cream on the third day. You know what? Two days later, when she finished her five-day fast, it was still a five-day fast. She had gotten all the benefits, and she felt great. Never toss away a phenomenal moment of personal success. Fasting is a superpower. Build yourself up with the right biohacks—what you eat, when you eat, how long you fast, how you sleep and exercise—and you will discover that you can do all sorts of crazy stuff. The superpower is already inside you, waiting to be set free. But you sure won't set it free by fixating on lists of calorie counts.

Every person reacts differently to fasting, based on his or her age, weight, and genetic predisposition. Still, there are predictable similarities in how the human metabolism reacts to a period of time without ingesting food. It's at this basic, biochemical level that intermittent fasting gives you totally different results from CICO diets. This is the origin point of your superpower and of all the biohacks that facilitate it. This is the microscopic pathway leading to your best self.

THE STAGES OF FASTING

STAGE ZERO OF FASTING BEGINS THE MOMENT YOU FINISH YOUR MEAL.

You can think of the time from a meal until three hours after that meal as "Stage Zero" of fasting, or as the anti-fast. This is a normal eating pattern for most of us: you eat breakfast; three hours later, you eat lunch; a few hours after that, you eat dinner. You will feel pretty normal at this stage, since your body is still busy digesting the last thing you ate. But even during the anti-fast, you can do things to help train yourself for fasting. The most obvious one is to avoid constant snacking between meals (especially snacking on the nasty processed foods that are lying around a lot of offices and homes). There's actually a lot going on between meals, and you want to get out of the way and let your metabolism do its thing.

In those immediate postmeal hours, your body is digesting the carbs, proteins, and fats from your food, turning them into amino acids, fatty acids, and above all, glucose. Your pancreas releases insulin, which will be used to transport all that new glucose into cells, where some of it will immediately be used to produce energy and protein synthesis in your muscles. This period of time is known as the growth period or anabolic period, since the nutrients your body needs are all readily available. *Anabolic* literally means "building up." Your body is drawing on the energy and raw materials from the digested food to build up the essential molecules in your body. Some of the surplus glucose will be combined with water and stored as glycogen, a starchlike molecule that is an efficient way to store energy, or turned into adipose tissue. Bad news: every molecule of glycogen carries two bloat-inducing molecules of water that effectively hide your abs. Those fitness models you see on magazines? They've all been fasting so they have no glycogen-water love handles.

This is also when your hunger hormones kick in. Ghrelin is the primary hunger hormone, activated to tell your body it's time to eat. Leptin is the antihunger hormone, which tells you when you're full. Ghrelin levels decline after a meal as leptin levels rise. CCK creates a short-lived sensation of fullness after eating and slows the emptying of the stomach to aid digestion.

A great many diet plans advise you to eat every three hours to keep your metabolism humming along at warp speed so you can lose weight. If you follow that advice, the minute you hit the three-hour mark and you start feeling the slightest bit hungry, you answer the ghrelin response and eat something. If you don't, cravings kick in, your blood sugar level starts to drop, and you yell at someone nearby because you feel like crap. (You are feeling hypogly-bitchy!) Your biggest question at three hours isn't whether to wait a few more hours before eating but what type of calories you'll be putting in your body for your next meal. This is a bad idea because your body never gets a break, and the constantly high blood sugar level created by constant snacking ages you.

If you feel hungry three or four hours after your last meal, it's because you ate kryptonite foods, you didn't eat good fats, you didn't eat enough, or your metabolism hasn't been trained to shift easily between burning sugars and burning fats—most likely all three. You have two choices: eat quickly, but do it so you will be satisfied for hours afterward, or face the music, experience some real discomfort, and fast anyway. Fasting after eating a meal is the hardest way to start a fast, and I don't recommend it. You already fast for eight hours every night, which is why starting a fast in the morning is easiest.

STAGE ONE OF FASTING KICKS IN FOUR TO SIXTEEN HOURS AFTER YOUR LAST MEAL.

This is the beginner's fast, or the 16:8 intermittent fast. Now you are beginning to break with the stereotypical three-meals-a-day eating pattern. There's an old adage that if you place a frog directly into a pot of boiling water, it will leap out immediately, but if you place it in warm water and then slowly turn up the heat, it will remain in the pot even as the water boils. This is an apt metaphor for the relationship between people and fasting. You are likely not ready, as a fasting beginner, to go even one full day without food. Do it too suddenly, without the right tools, and you may find yourself dreaming of eating that frog before you give up on fasting entirely. Given enough time, though, a daylong fast is not difficult at all. You just have to turn up the heat slowly.

The whole intermittent fasting process begins in this four- to sixteen-hour window. All the energy coursing through your body after a meal has been put to use. Now the body switches over to stored energy. Glucose is still the prime fuel, though now you are tapping it in the form of glycogen, which has to be pulled from your muscles or your liver.

Skipping breakfast will get you through the three hours after dinner, a night of good sleep, and up to 11:00 a.m. before breaking your fast for real at midmorning. This is known as 16:8 intermittent fasting (sixteen hours without a meal, then an eight-hour eating window before starting the cycle again). It is one of the most common rhythms of intermittent fasting. There are a lot of chemical changes happening inside you at this point.

During a 16:8 fast, your blood glucose levels drop, leading to a decrease in insulin secretion in the pancreas. You may begin to experience the sensations of hunger, light-headedness, and agitation that often accompany low blood sugar, especially if you have never fasted before. After twelve hours without food, your blood glucose level will have dropped by about 20 percent. The hormone known as glucagon is secreted to activate glycogen breakdown, which provides more glucose. As your body starts to use up the glycogen in your muscles, the body starts releasing adrenaline and cortisol, which free up extra energy from the protein in your body for emergencies. You will need less sleep and feel extra energy, though it's possible you will also feel somewhat cranky.

Once you master the Stage One fast, you're going to realize that you're just not hungry at 11:00 a.m. anymore. The gnawing feeling is gone. A colleague can put bagels right in front of you at work and you won't have to fight the urge to snatch one. You simply won't crave them. Most people who practice Stage One 16:8 intermittent fasting several days a week for a month find it easy to extend to advanced Stage One, in which you eat an entire day's worth of food in two meals between about 2:00 and 8:00 p.m.

STAGE TWO OF FASTING IS THE ONE-MEAL-A-DAY FAST, OFTEN ABBREVIATED AS OMAD.

Once you pass the sixteen-hour mark, your body realizes there is very little glucose to be found and begins the full transition to fat burning. Doing so sets into motion a complex interaction of hormones and chemicals that enable your body to use fat as a fuel source, a key step in training your body to be metabolically flexible.

Technically, OMAD is just a twenty-four-hour fast: you have a meal, and you don't eat until you have a meal at the same time the next day. Calling it OMAD somehow gives it a little more attitude, like a fast with tattoos and cool hair. The abbreviation sounds like "nomad." If calling your twenty-four-hour fast OMAD makes you feel good, then go with OMAD. It's kind of sexy to say, "I'm OMAD today." You can do the Zoolander hair flip for added effect.

A twenty-four-hour fast causes the body to activate lipolysis, a process in the liver that breaks down fat molecules into fatty acids. This act of chemical transformation is regulated by a protein known as peroxisome proliferator-activated receptor-alpha, or PPAR-alpha, which activates the key genetic mechanisms needed to create, transport, and consume fatty acids. The fatty acids, in turn, are transformed into energy-rich ketones (technically, into *ketone bodies*) through a process known as beta-oxidation. There are three different types of ketones: acetone, acetoacetate, and beta-hydroxybutyrate, or BHB. They are all important to ketosis, the state in which your body is running on fat. Finally, the liver launches the ketones into the bloodstream. This state of ketosis occurs more quickly if you have already burned muscle glycogen earlier in the fast through exercise, which is why exercise is an important aspect of biohacking your fast. You'll hear a lot more about this later.

Along with these chemical changes, your heart rate and blood pressure drop as your body switches into energy-saving mode. Overall, your basal metabolic rate, or BMR, becomes lower and more efficient. There has been a lot of recent scientific interest in the effects of OMAD fasting but so far only a small number of published, controlled studies. One of them, conducted by a group led by David J. Baer at the US Department of Agriculture, found lower levels of triglycerides and higher levels of HDL ("good") cholesterol in the blood of healthy middle-aged adults who reduced the frequency of their meals.[3]

OMAD is a cornerstone of my intermittent fasting regimen, and it should be for yours, too. You might be surprised, then, by what I'm going to tell you next: doing OMAD every day is a terrible idea. Fasting purists get their hackles up when they hear that, but after ten years of answering people's questions about fasting on my blog, I've lost track of the number of people who feel great on OMAD-style intermittent fasting, vow to do it every day, and regret their decision two to four months later when they have to climb out of a health hole they dug for themselves. *Intermittent means intermittent!* If you do OMAD every day, expect to see your sex hormone levels fall (this applies to both men and women), your sleep quality drop, and your hair thin. People over thirty-five usually feel these effects before younger fasters, but they are almost inevitable at some point.

For maximum impact, I recommend regularly changing not only the duration of your fast but also the style. You might try a high-protein breakfast with plenty of fat on Monday, OMAD on Tuesday, intermittent fasting on Wednesday, OMAD on Thursday, intermittent fasting on Friday. On Saturday you eat whatever the heck you want, then on Sunday you circle back to OMAD. You are making your body stronger by cycling into and out of lipolysis and ketosis. Typically, you would do your twenty-four-hour fasts by eating dinner only. But if you can, challenge yourself and skip dinner occasionally. When you eat again, it will be about thirty-six hours since your last meal, and you'll push into the next stage of fasting.

STAGE THREE OF FASTING (36 TO 120 HOURS) IS A MORE ADVANCED TECHNIQUE FOR PEOPLE WHO ALREADY KNOW HOW TO DO SHORTER FASTS SAFELY AND COMFORTABLY.

Let's say you just went thirty-six hours, because you slept before you ate again. If you haven't done an extended fast before, it's hard to believe that this is even possible. But by the time you get here, you will learn that it's not that hard. In fact, thirty-six hours is my favorite fast.

After twenty-four hours, ketones are your primary fuel source: you are fully in ketosis. But the brain runs on glucose, not ketones, so a process known as gluconeogenesis occurs. The body ingeniously turns fat, ketones, and amino acids into glucose—sometimes producing as much as 80 grams per day—keeping your mind sharp.

At a time when you might expect your hunger to be at an all-time high, your production of ghrelin hormone drops off, so you actually cease to experience hunger pangs. As your body taps into its fat reserves, it also clears out the toxins that are often stored along with the fat molecules. Your body is pumped by the changes in your metabolism and is screaming at you to keep going. If you're feeling inspired, you could easily skip another couple of meals before breaking your fast. When you hit the thirty-six-hour mark and make the bold choice to go for two complete days without food, you'll hear your body asking, "Is it actually possible that I can go forty-eight hours without food? I think I can do it."

The thirty-six-hour fast is my favorite because it is vanishingly easy. I go to sleep (that's eight hours of fasting), then have Bulletproof Coffee for breakfast so my energy is high and my blood sugar is low.

Lunchtime rolls around, and I'm not hungry. I tell myself I might have dinner, which makes my body stop thinking about food. But at dinner, I tell myself, "Hey, skip dinner and sleep on it, and you'll get another eight hours of fasting—that will be thirty-two hours!" When I wake up, I find that I don't even want breakfast. I have no hunger at all. By the time I eat lunch, I really only had to skip one meal: dinner the night before. A thirty-six-hour fast without feeling denied or even very hungry is entirely possible.

Still feeling good? You may be ready to keep your fast going up to 120 hours—five days, or a full workweek. This is an advanced level that can take you into a spiritual fast (we will discuss this idea in more detail in chapter 7), but you should approach this with caution and only after you have become experienced with fasting.

At this point, most people enter a full state of ketosis, in which your body is breaking down its own fat for energy. It will also break down small amounts of muscle to turn into glucose through a process called gluconeogenesis. Some long-term keto dieters say that this is a great state to be in, and it is for a little while. Your body will break down old proteins first! The problem is that it's biologically difficult to turn protein into glucose, and you don't want to be doing it for long periods of time.

By now, your body has entered prolonged fasting mode. You will feel less mentally grounded but bursting with energy. If you get a hunger pain, have some water with a dash of sea salt in it or coffee or tea. It will pass quickly. Your levels of glucose and insulin have dropped for an extended period, decreasing your risk of metabolic disease. Meanwhile, your cells have become more resistant to toxins and stress. Your ghrelin production continues to drop, eliminating your sensation of hunger. Your ketone production increases as the body's demand for ketones rises. A pleasant by-product of this change is that ketones also help suppress ghrelin levels. This is not the painful fast you feared.

There are significant health benefits to these extended fasts. Your body will turn up autophagy, the recycling of cells, mitochondria, and cellular junk. Your liver will reduce its secretion of insulin-like growth factor 1, or IGF-1, a hormone that is structurally similar to insulin.

Although IGF-1 is crucial to normal bodily functioning, elevated levels are associated with cancer. But you need to pay attention when coming out of an extended fast: if you've fasted for several days or a week, the meal you choose to break the fast should include protein, fat, vegetables (carbohydrates), and lots of fiber. This combination will allow you to strike a good metabolic balance while keeping your gut bacteria healthy.

STAGE FOUR OF FASTING MAY SOUND IMPROBABLE TO ANYONE WHO HAS NEVER DONE IT BEFORE.

A fast that lasts more than 120 hours, or five days? Really? Yes, it is possible to live in ketosis for an extended period of time, if you are extremely attentive to your body's needs.

At this point, you've entered the outer zone of fasting. Anytime you fast more than 120 hours, you are almost guaranteed to lose weight unless you have some really serious metabolic issues. There is a problem that comes with that weight loss: when you shed a lot of fat quickly, the toxins in your body—the ones from Big Food and Mother Nature, the heavy metals, the pesticides, the mold toxins that are stored in your fat—are all released at the same time. In response, you will get headaches, you will feel groggy, and you will yell at people. Be psychologically prepared for that.

During Stage Four fasting, you will enter a kind of altered state in which your body has switched over to burning only fat. People often describe a "fasting high" in response to this new metabolic reality of complete ketosis. You likely won't need Bulletproof Coffee this far into a fast—your own inner furnace will be making ketones at full speed. It's a good idea to have some quiet time. Most people can't focus on really demanding tasks during a fast this long unless they're quite well trained in fasting.

Your glucose, insulin, and IGF-1 levels have gone way down by this point. You have broken away from the cycle of insulin resistance, which could help fend off diabetes. Your appetite is suppressed to a low level, even as your body's total energy expenditure remains steady.

You don't feel hungry, and you don't feel weak, either. Autophagy is in full swing in your body, clearing out toxins and dead cell parts. Your mitochondria are working more efficiently, so they are releasing fewer of the reactive, destructive charged molecules known as free radicals. Elevated levels of NAD+ in your bloodstream help retard the continuous oxidizing of your cells. These mechanisms all have an antiaging effect.

Despite these benefits, you should be wary of trying a Stage Four fast. Some studies have shown that ultralong fasts can be beneficial for hypertension[4] and may amplify the effectiveness of chemotherapy for cancer patients,[5] but extreme fasting can be quite dangerous or even fatal. It can weaken the heart, suppress the immune system, and lower blood pressure.

Detoxing during long fasts is extremely important because of all those compounds set free during weight loss; I recommend taking activated charcoal to help with your detox. You also want to take supplements to maintain your electrolytes: calcium, magnesium, potassium, and sodium in particular. That's especially important if you are doing a water fast or drinking just coffee and tea. You can get sick enough to require hospitalization if your electrolyte levels fall too low during a long fast. It's a good idea to have a doctor supervise any fast that runs ten days or longer. I don't recommend exercising during long fasts.

IN PRAISE OF INCONSISTENCY

You will notice that each stage of fasting affects the body in different ways and confers its own distinct benefits. That's part of the reason why it is good to mix up your fasting styles. Some days, you just might realize that you don't have the energy reserves to fast as long as you wanted. That's okay, too.

Still, it's human nature to think, hey, if something is good, surely more of it must be better! If you do an OMAD fast, you will feel great. You will feel strong. So why *not* do OMAD every day? Think about it this way: a piece of cheesecake is good, right? (If you're not a fan of cheesecake, just substitute something else you love and roll with me here.) What about two pieces—even better? Uh . . . maybe. Now you are being served your third piece, and you might be starting to think, "Whoa, that's a bit much, but I suppose I can try." Four pieces, and you're like, "Please stop." But no, no, no! You said that more was good. You have to eat it.

You get the idea. People do this with vegan diets, they do it with keto, and they do it with fasting. It's possible to get hooked on fasting, just as you can get hooked on any other style of dieting. I call it the "fasting trap" (see chapter 10 for more detail on this). Straight up, the vast majority of people will break themselves if they do OMAD all the time. You'll feel great for a while, but then you'll realize, "Something's not right." If you're a woman, your cycle will feel off. If you're a guy, you won't feel your usual morning kickstand. These are signs that you overdid it. That's why I recommend cycles of intermittent fasting: different cycles of fasting, along with breaks from fasting entirely.

Dieting books and fasting guides love to load you up with rules. Here's what they almost never tell you: *The body loves consistency because it needs to do less work to survive in a consistent world.* The trouble is, when the body does less work, it gets lazy. If you send a signal to your body that the world is *not* consistent, it will rebuild itself to thrive in that world. That's why your body will be much stronger if you deny it consistency: you will build yourself up by challenging yourself.

Natural selection exerts a tremendous evolutionary pressure on every creature to take in as much food as possible and expend as little energy as possible. Your brain, your body, the quadrillions of cells inside you, and even the ancient bacteria that merged with animal cells a couple billion years ago—they're all telling you the same thing: Sit on the couch. Have a bag of chips or whatever other source of calories you come across. That's what they're programmed to do, and that's what they will do over and over if you allow them to by leaving them in a consistent environment.

But if you introduce a change in behavior or resources, your cells are forced to become more resilient. Long ago, you might have needed resilience so that you could leap up from your sleep and make a sudden sprint away from a predator. Your body had to be strong enough and flexible enough to do that, or you wouldn't survive. Today, things are a bit different: You can adjust the types of foods you eat and when you eat them and make your cells more resilient that way. Dietary exercise is exactly analogous to physical exercise. Long periods of in-action are terrible for your health; long periods of dietary consistency are similarly terrible for your metabolic health. It's one more reason that rigid, CICO-style dieting is such a bad idea.

The more you mix things up and the more you reject consistency, the stronger and more flexible your cells will be. They will treat every day as a day when you are ready to leap into action. They will be ready to extract energy from any kind of food. They will no longer be trained to crave one particular snack or comfort food.

By reading this book, you have already started making a sincere effort to embrace inconsistency and free yourself from your cravings. The last thing you want to do now is imprison yourself with a new kind of craving, a craving for a certain style of fasting. You need to give yourself breaks and mix things up. You may reach the point where you think, "I don't want to eat carbs. I don't like how I feel when I eat carbs. Never again." The correct response to that is "Shut up and eat some carbs from time to time." Sure, you don't want to eat processed sugar. I'm not encouraging you to gorge on cotton candy and Tootsie Rolls. But you can have a sweet potato or some rice. Or even some dairy-free ice cream. You'll be okay. You'll be more than okay, in fact, because you'll be teaching your body to stay metabolically flexible.

You don't want to be locked up by the fasting police any more than you want to be locked up by the calorie police. Fortunately, intermittent fasting is inherently flexible. As impossible as it might seem right now, you are capable of fasting for any length of time you attempt. Once you master the easy stages, you can try out the longer, more challenging ones. Over time, you will come to appreciate the different feelings and the different benefits you get from each of them. Always talk to your doctor before you embark on an extended fast, and stop a fast early if you start to feel really unwell, especially on the longer ones.

Believe it or not, we haven't even gotten to one of the most sweep-ing benefits of intermittent fasting, which will liberate you from some-thing you probably aren't even aware is holding you back—although it almost certainly is. Read on.

4

FAST FOR LONG LIFE

Even before entering the cave for my vision quest, I felt like I'd arrived at a special place. From the outside, it looked as if the forces of nature had conspired to sculpt the perfect Instagram shot, with millions of years of geology and erosion coming together in this moment (except that Mother Nature probably hates Instagram). The gorgeous red-rock formation let sunlight in through a large, spherical portal in one wall that overlooked the valley below. There was a feather on the ground near the opening of the cave, lying there like a talisman. I instinctively picked it up, saw how it reflected the sunlight, and attached it to my backpack. At the end of the quest, I learned it was a bald eagle feather. I had no idea at the time—it's actually illegal to possess a bald eagle feather, unless you're from an indigenous tribe—but an eagle feather is believed to carry extra spiritual significance during a vision quest. To many of the local peoples, the eagle is a symbol of wisdom and courage, and an eagle feather can be used as a tool for healing. However it got there, I was grateful to have found it and gave it to Delilah on my return.

Yet even with all of those apparent synchronicities lining up the way you'd expect in a movie, a voice in my head nagged at me. A vision quest is not about bathing in glittering light and waving feathers around; it is about doing hard physical and spiritual work. I had come here to be hungry and alone and to forge myself into something stronger. I felt a nagging desire to go to a different cave, with no one around for miles. But apparently, that was not what fate had in store for me. The best I could do was to let things happen as they were going to happen and make the most of the situation by honoring Delilah's instructions to remain in silence.

I chose a relatively flat, peaceful spot in the cave where I could sit alone(ish) for hours and then set up my sleeping bag, practicing complete silence (almost) the whole while. Despite my best efforts, I could hear my stomach and my brain grumbling about how hungry I was. I felt famished all day and night, but I did my best to confront and conquer those cravings. That first night, I fantasized about packing up my stuff and hiking to another cave that Delilah had mentioned was a mile away. There, I thought, I could truly face hunger by myself.

The next morning, when I dutifully turned on my phone to compose the text confirming that I was safe, it buzzed with a new incoming message from the shaman. "Pack up your stuff and come to the trailhead at 8am," Delilah had texted. "I'm going to take you to another cave." She hadn't been kidding when she'd said she would be watching us remotely.

I hiked to the trailhead, and Delilah pulled up in her old pickup. Then she said something that blew my mind: "Last night you were thinking you really wanted to go to the First Woman cave, and that's where you want to do your vision quest. So here I am to pick you up and take you there."

According to tradition, true shamans can read your inner wants and desires, but I had never seen that ability in action. I hadn't said a word to her, and I like to think I have a pretty good poker face. It was just one of several improbable-seeming things that happened during the vision quest. There are lots of hypotheses about intuitives and enough well-constructed scientific studies to hint that some people can accurately perceive other people's thoughts. Maybe Delilah had noticed a tiny, subconscious hesitation in me while we'd been on our way to the original cave. Maybe she really could tune in to my energy from afar. The first step of the scientific method is to observe, so I can only tell you that that was what happened.

I refuse to fall into the trap that has held science back so often: the trap of facing evidence but then saying, "I don't believe that could happen, therefore it didn't happen." If you start out insisting that something's impossible, you will dismiss the evidence of it. In the process, you might miss something vital that could change the way you look at the world.

Call it freethinking or call it scientific method; either way, you'll live a better life if you allow yourself to observe without prejudice or preconception. There's a lot of evidence that your body won't starve or even be harmed if you go a few days—or even weeks—without food. You may find that hard to believe. There's an enormous food industry that doesn't want you to believe that, and your body has been well trained not to believe it—just as my mind didn't want to believe that the shaman could know what I had been dreaming about. But when you set aside your beliefs and open yourself up to new experiences, incredible things can happen.

EVOLVED TO EAT—BUT NOT LIKE THIS

The history of human evolution is also the history of food. Believe it or not, it's the history of fasting, too. Our bodies and brains are inherently adapted to it.

The earliest fossil evidence of *Homo sapiens* pinpoints that our species originated roughly 300,000 years ago. Three meals a day were hardly the norm during that time. Our ancestors were opportunistic eaters, but above all they were hunters and gatherers, roaming the African plains in search of wild game:[1] gazelles, antelope, wildebeests, zebras, and buffalos, with plants as backup. They traveled as clans, often walking miles at a time to find their prey. High speed was not as important as endurance or intelligence, because animals are inherently better sprinters. When an antelope or gazelle or whatever animal was finally caught, the feast was shared by all. There was rarely enough meat to last more than a few days.

When the food was exhausted, they hunted for more and subsisted on the few edible plants that would have been in season and not too toxic to eat. Until the next meal could be run down, everyone went hungry, yet no one died from going a few days without food. Fasting— either with no food or with a vanishingly few calories from plants— was simply a part of our ancestors' lifestyles. They had no choice. This habit of eating and then fasting continued for not just for decades or centuries or even a few millennia; humans have lived a lifestyle of feasting and fasting for almost 290,000 years. The fasting lifestyle is far more ancient than that, even; it's the way of life for most large carnivores. Lions don't sit down to three meals a day, for instance. When they get a good catch, they eat; then they may go three or four days before another major meal.

You may have heard about the "carnivore diet," which combines a diet of only grass-fed meat with intermittent fasting. The good news about the carnivore diet is that it contains none of the plant toxins that spike hunger, which makes fasting really easy. Think of the carnivore diet as simply fasting from vegetables. If you're like most people who try it, you'll do it for a few weeks, love how you feel, and then eat a kryptonite-free salad. You'll also gain a new understanding of how good you feel when you remove things that cause problems. Full fasting simply removes all foods that could be causing your bloat, brain fog, and metabolic problems. If you do it, follow the rules: eat only animals that are grass fed or wild caught, and eat the whole animal, including organs and connective tissues for collagen. As I said, intermittent fasting works with *every* diet under the sun.

One critical factor that distinguishes humans from other carnivores is that we use tools—especially fire. Modern genetic studies indicate that the invention of cooking was critically important in unlocking nutrition from foods that were too tough or too toxic to eat without being roasted over a flame. Cooking also makes it possible to consume more parts of an animal and to eat meat with less chewing. Scientists have found physical evidence of cooking hearths that are 500,000 years old; the Harvard anthropologist Richard Wrangham argues that our ancestors might have begun cooking nearly 2 million years ago.[2] Either way, cooking is so ancient that it predates *Homo sapiens.* In retrospect, I wish I'd known that when I spent almost a year making myself sick on a raw vegan diet!

Our ability to get more energy and fat into the body allowed us to evolve bigger brains than those of other species. A bigger brain requires more electricity running through the body. Although your brain makes up just 2 percent of your weight, it consumes 15 to 20 percent of your metabolic energy. It takes a lot of electrons to power the 100 billion or so cells inside our mental supercomputer.

A big brain is the secret to our species' evolutionary success, because it allowed our ancestors to think their way out of problems. It does the same thing for you, too—if you use it well. While some of our competitors evolved a thicker skull or bigger claws or a longer neck so they could eat leaves from tall trees, we got the big brain. Language, culture, science, technology, large-scale cooperation, and planning for the future are all by-products of this change. We humans are the dominant species of life on Earth today because of the size and complexity of our brain.

One of the big brain's greatest contributions was that it allowed us to think our way out of starvation. Even after the introduction of spears, nets, and bows and arrows for hunting, humankind continued to fast. Not only did we thrive, but our brain thrived as well. The average brain size of early humans kept getting bigger and bigger, with much of the expansion happening in the section known as the prefrontal cortex. Over many tens of thousands of years, this lobe right behind our forehead developed into a powerhouse of decision making, planning, cognitive behavior, social interaction, and personality.

The act of fasting did not diminish the body's evolutionary adaptations. Instead, it encouraged them. In effect, we became smarter by not eating for a while and *then* eating fatty animal foods to power our brains. You may feel panic if your next meal is more than six hours away, but your body knows better. When you don't eat for a while, the brain simply switches from running on glucose to running on ketones. The switchover, which can occur as soon as you go fourteen hours without consuming food, but most often in twenty-four to forty-eight hours, happens automatically and almost imperceptibly—at least it does once your metabolism becomes accustomed to this type of switching. When you're new to burning fat, the switch takes two to four days, and in the meantime, you don't feel great. This book contains the things you need to know to skip that painful process. They are things our caveman ancestors simply didn't have access to because they didn't have the ability to modify their food that we do.

Fasting unleashes your hidden evolutionary powers. Ketones have more electrons per gram—more raw energy density—than glucose. When you pour ketones into your cells, it's as if you went to the gas station and put in high-octane racing gasoline. Because fat has more calories per gram than sugar, your body can metabolize ketones to produce more heat per gram than glucose. Mixing metaphors: eating fat instead of sugar is like drinking a vodka instead of a beer (although in this case, it's okay to drink and drive!). It has a different effect on you, because it is so much more potent.

There's a reason animals fast when they get injured. Whether you realize it or not, humans do this, too. The last time you were really sick, did you have an appetite? Our body naturally reduces our need for food when we're ill, allowing it to spend its energy on repair rather than digestion and heal itself without the presence of toxins. The same thing happens when you take long breaks between meals. Fasting activates a built-in adaptive healing process.

Think about that the next time you fear dying if you miss lunch.

THREE MEALS A DAY? WHY?

After cooking, the next revolutionary change in the human diet occurred roughly 10,000 years ago, when *Homo sapiens* learned how to farm. Instead of roaming the savanna on foot, searching for meals, and eating with large breaks between unpredictably timed meals, we became tied to the land and to our herds of domesticated animals. We became anchored to one location, because if we left that would mean the end of our farm. The villages that grew around farms needed workers for various jobs, and soon we stopped moving and started sitting a lot more. After more than a quarter of a million years of routine fasting, the new food supply that we grew on small plots of land meant we could eat a meal a day, every day. Then as we got better at agriculture, it was possible to plan on two meals. The modern routine of breakfast, lunch, and dinner is less than two centuries old.[3] Later on, we added nachos and potato chips in between those meals, while watching television.

Abundant food should have made it possible for all of us to be creative geniuses. Perhaps those early farmers also planted the seed for CICO diets because they swapped meat and fat calories from animals for abundant amounts of carbohydrates from plants. In one fell swoop, they killed fasting and replaced the highest-nutrient foods with corn and wheat. This is a great system, at least if you're one of the lucky few at the top. All those dull minds could toil in the field, which freed the elites to explore arts, science, and chemistry and also get the best, most expensive food—from grass-fed animals, instead of having to spend the day hunting. But if you were one of the majority working in the fields, you led a dull, nutrient-deficient life. The new diet even led to a decline in the average height of humans, because much of the time we were at war with our own biology.

Starting in the early nineteenth century, with the advent of the Industrial Revolution, people in the Western world all began eating more or less on the same schedule. Before that, the concept of time wasn't as regimented. You didn't need to know exactly what hour of the day it was; farmers just cared about when the sun rose and set. After the Industrial Revolution, though, a pocket watch became an incredibly valuable item, because it told you when the trains were going to arrive and depart. Trains ran on precise schedules. Then factories and stores ran on precise schedules. Our new connection to time, which was driven largely by train schedules, led us to start planning our meals for specific times each day. We scheduled our food around trains, not our actual hunger or the needs of our bodies.

Let's go back to that metaphor of putting gas in your car. What if someone told you that you would have to drive to the gas station every Tuesday and Thursday at 3:00 p.m. to put ten gallons of gas into your car. Why? There's no explanation; you just know that everybody does it, so it must be the normal thing to do. It doesn't matter where and when or how much you have driven your car. It doesn't even matter if your tank is empty or full. Every Tuesday and Thursday at 3:00 p.m., you fill the tank. That's just the way it is.

Sometimes you go to the gas station, put the nozzle in, and the tank is already full. You always buy ten gallons, though, so you just pump the gas onto the ground or maybe put it into a separate little storage can in the trunk. Huh, this is getting weird. Still, there must be a reason it's the tradition, right? Pretty soon your car is full of extra gas in the trunk that you don't need. Now you've got junk in your trunk, you might say. Eating the same-size meal at the same time every day makes no rational sense, no more than filling your car with gas on that nutty schedule does. If you're not careful, it really will put junk in your trunk. But it's tradition, so we generally go along without even thinking about it.

A lot of our weird attitudes about food have emerged from the clash between our evolutionary origins and our modern cultural traditions. Eating is essential to survival, yet it isn't only a biological imperative; it's a sensual experience and a communal ritual. Cooking for and feeding one another is an intimate act, a spiritual act. It relieves stress even as it puts fuel and nutrients into your body. Our big brains need lots of energy, but they also need periods of fasting and regeneration. On the other hand, the social structures and the food industry created by our big brains keep telling us to eat regular meals—to eat whether or not we're hungry—so we keep craving food all the time.

But as we know, in addition to energy and nutrients, food fills you with toxins. We learned to focus on satisfying our energy needs above all else, because that was (and is) how we stayed alive. Next we learned to focus on flavor, because a good taste was (and sometimes still is) an indicator that a food was nutritious and high quality. But we've never really learned how to avoid toxins, unless they kill us or disable us quickly. The subtle, slow-working toxins in food are difficult to recognize. And frankly, for almost all of history, when faced with the choice between famine and eating food that has calories along with some toxins, we have rationally chosen to take the hit from the toxins. Sometimes they even taste good!

One surprising example is rice. Brown rice has more calories and fiber than white rice, but in the countries where rice is a historical part of the diet, people always ate white rice when they could afford it. Brown rice was long considered peasant food. Why? Everyone knew that they didn't feel as good when they ate brown rice because it's hard on the gut. Today, we know it contains lectins, those nasty plant toxins that keep animals from eating rice, and about eighty times as much arsenic as is found in white rice. That's why white rice exists: it was milled to get rid of the toxins in the husk. Then modern science stepped in and ignored the toxins, instead praising the extra fiber and nominal amounts of vitamins in the rice husks. Health food experts told us to eat brown rice because it has more good stuff in it. The hidden cost in gut irritation from lectins, arsenic poisoning, and cravings wasn't in the equation. After you eat brown rice, do you notice a "food baby"—a little swelling in your stomach?

Whenever you experience inflammation, it means that some electrons that were supposed to power your body instead went into inflammation. Your body will want you to eat more to make up for the lost electrons. Try it yourself. Brown rice keeps you full for a little longer because it is hard to digest, but after that, big cravings come. White rice is digested quickly but without the cravings. Our ancestors knew that the extra nutrients in brown rice aren't worth the trouble that comes with the toxins you get. If you think rice is confusing, just ponder all of the sensory overload and conflicting information that hits you when you're walking down the aisles of the supermarket. Your poor brain wasn't evolved to handle this.

Your brain says: the most important thing is to make sure I get tons of energy, because I might not get another meal. That weird visceral programming happens before you have a chance to think about it, unless you bring your brain back to its baseline through fasting.

Or let's use another example: a cookie. Your body has an automated system to make sure that you never, ever run out of energy. If you could somehow take control of the automated system and make it consciously visible—if you could look at the cookie like Neo from *The Matrix*, seeing the zeros and ones that represent your body's operating system—you would see that the cookie contains lots of energy. Do you need energy right now? Perhaps not, but your brain knows that the energy will make you feel good. Does the cookie have nutrients in it? Maybe, maybe not, but that's okay. You can take a supplement if you want nutrients, and some of the other foods you eat will probably balance it out. Even if you have a very basic supplement budget, you're not going to run out of nutrients.

But does the cookie also have toxins in it? Your brain has no idea, and unless you've read and decoded the ingredients (or made the cookie yourself), you probably have no idea, either. In the absence of information, the evolution-honed message you get from your brain is: go ahead, eat. What you're going to find very quickly is that your body tells you to eat everything, including foods that are full of toxins and things that have more energy than you actually need. And the toxins themselves cause more food cravings when they slow down your mitochondria.

You're left asking yourself, "Why does my body want me to eat that cookie?" It's not a rational impulse. In fact, it's fueled largely by emotion. Remember, we all want to feel safe. We all want to feel loved. There isn't a better way to feel loved and safe than to be a baby nursing on your mother's chest. That wiring is still in there, hidden beneath your thoughts. No wonder fasting pushes your buttons.

We all have an emotional association with food. Some of us take it a step further by using food as a form of comfort or a passionate connection. That's one reason why I ended up in the cave. I wanted to make sure I dealt with my emotional attachments to food as a part of my journey. I wanted to completely understand why the hell I kept putting food into my mouth, even when I knew I didn't want or need it, even when my body was distorted by stretch marks. These kinds of revelations are not easy for me to write about, and I'm sure they're not easy for you to think about, but they're real. You must confront them in order to embrace them and, ultimately, free yourself from them.

Nourishing someone is an intimate act. Nourishing *yourself* is an intimate act. You're literally taking something from the environment, putting it inside you, and absorbing fuel, nutrients, and toxins from your digestive tract to make that food become part of your body. As humans, we have all kinds of emotional baggage connected to the act of eating. Most of it is preconscious, because each cell in your body wants you to eat, independent of you actually wanting to eat. In the modern world, food is so abundant that the want can be activated all the time—unless you train yourself to activate the feeling of *going without* while still feeling safe and loved.

You are constantly hearing a dialogue between your biology saying that if you don't eat, you'll die, and your adult, conscious, evolved human brain saying that it needs food to feel safe. But you don't have to listen. Keep telling yourself: neither message is true.

THE PRICE OF PLENTY

The modern era of abundant food means that much of the world no longer has to worry about the famine and starvation that threatened our species through most of its history. All of this plenty comes with a significant trade-off, however, in our loss of fasting and all of the benefits it provides.

Mark Mattson, a neuroscientist at Johns Hopkins University and the former head of the Laboratory of Neurosciences at the National Institute on Aging, summed up this dilemma in a 2014 review article, "Challenging Oneself Intermittently to Improve Health." He came to largely the same conclusions that I did in the cave. "As a consequence of the modern 'couch potato' lifestyle, signaling pathways that mediate beneficial effects of environmental challenges on health and disease resistance are disengaged," he wrote. ". . . Reversal of the epidemic of diseases caused by unchallenging lifestyles will require a society-wide effort to re-introduce intermittent fasting, exercise, and consumption of plants."[4]

In the early days of agriculture, crowded working conditions and proximity to domesticated animals, as well as concentrated human waste in villages, ushered in an unprecedented number of deaths from parasites and infectious diseases. The list included many of the diseases that show up in the earliest recorded history, such as cholera, typhoid, leprosy, smallpox, malaria, tuberculosis, and herpes. We passed diseases to our animals, and in time they gave them right back to us. In due course, *Homo sapiens* traveled away from Africa into the land we now call Europe, where they interbred with the closely related Neanderthals who had already migrated there. The two shared diseases, and there is some evidence that the infections we carried helped wipe out the Neanderthals.

Early farmers didn't eat at the same time every day. It took factories, trains, and the Industrial Revolution to regiment our eating habits. Until we started eating three meals a day, the chances of dying of high blood pressure, insulin resistance, heart attack, and cancer were significantly less than they are today. Overeating and obesity were almost nonexistent for thousands upon thousands of years. Nowadays they qualify as global pandemics in their own right. Cardiovascular disease kills an estimated 18 million people a year. More than 400 million people worldwide suffer from diabetes, according to the World Health Organization.[5]

Intermittent fasting is a way to restore balance. It can set your evolutionary self into harmony with your modern self, easing the tension inside you.

I often find it funny that so many people regard intermittent fasting as a new and controversial idea. It's more like a deep human wisdom that we've lost and now need to recover. The practice of deliberate fasting dates back thousands of years and has long been associated with wellness, longevity, and personal growth rather than mere denial. Fasting is a central element of Ayurveda, the system of health developed in India three thousand years ago. The ancient Greek philosopher Pythagoras used fasting as a path to enlightenment, reportedly requiring his students to fast for forty days before their exams. Paracelsus, a sixteenth-century Swiss physician who was a leader in the medical revolution of the Renaissance, proclaimed fasting to be "the physician within." In the late 1800s, the American physician Edward H. Dewey tried to revive these ideas by promoting a fast-based "no-breakfast plan" in his wildly popular book *The True Science of Living*. He claimed that nearly every modern disease is caused by "more or less habitual eating in excess."[6] Yup.

The story is the same among many indigenous American cultures. Native American tribes practiced fasting in both private and public ceremonies. In some First Nations tribes, this process began at puberty, with a solitary time of fasting and praying that lasted from one to four days. For adults, fasting preceded important events such as hunting or war. There were even occasions when entire tribes would fast together to enhance their sense of community. One Cherokee spiritual leader explained fasting "as a means to spiritualize the human nature and quicken the spiritual vision by abstinence from earthly food."[7]

Over the course of history, almost every world religion has made a similar connection to fasting as a means of enhancing spiritual development. The Christian, Jewish, Muslim, Buddhist, and Hindu faiths all advocate a period of fasting to attain spiritual enlightenment. In the Old Testament, Moses and Daniel fasted to enrich their faith. Later on, Jesus would fast forty days and nights in the desert. Traditionally, Catholics fasted from meat on Ash Wednesday and Good Friday and often at other times during Lent. Jews fast on Yom Kippur as a way to reset their relationship with their community and with God. The Muslim holy month of Ramadan has fasting as one of its cornerstones, with the faithful abstaining from all food and drink between dawn and dusk.

Across the religious spectrum, many orders of monks enhance their already ascetic lifestyle by eating nothing after noon each day. Memorably, Mohandas Gandhi fasted for political reasons on at least fourteen different occasions, with three of the fasts lasting at least twenty-one days each. At those times, he lived on nothing but water and salt. "What the eyes are for the outer world," he said, "fasts are for the inner."

It makes sense that a highly evolved brain, freed from preoccupation with obtaining food and fueled by energy-rich ketones, would be primed to explore the highest aspect of its cognitive powers. But the spiritual side of fasting did not lend itself readily to scientific investigation until recent improvements in neuroscience. Even without electrodes, anyone experienced in meditation and fasting will attest that different levels of consciousness are much easier to attain when fasting. One of those elevated levels is called Samadhi. In Hindu yoga, Samadhi is a deep level of ecstasy and superconscious perception in which people feel themselves become one with the entire universe, merging into God. Fasting expedites this process.

In other words, I wasn't being a kook when I decided to go into a cave and immerse myself in a fast. Sages all through history have done similar things in their search for enlightenment and self-realization. I may not be anywhere near the level of history's great sages, but sitting in a cave and fasting really does work. How much of it was the physical environment of the cave, how much of it was the solitude, and how much of it was the fasting? That I can't tell you, but I definitely walked out of that experience a changed man.

So why do so few people fast today, except as part of a religious ritual (or as part of a miserable, calorie-counting diet built around self-denial)? Mostly it's because of the horrible emotions and feelings associated with fasting, especially with the first stages of fasting. You can blame that on your ancestors—or rather, on the evolutionary processes that shaped them. Despite the ready abundance of food in the modern developed world, there is a signaling process built into your brain that says, "Don't fast, because fasting equals danger and fasting equals pain."

Here is a message for you to send back to your brain: "That's bullshit."

It's as important for you to fast as it is to eat a meal. Sounds insane, right? You have to eat in order to live. But you also have to fast in order to live well. Eating is effortless, but the ability to complete a fast is also effortless once you learn the skills and the mind-sets in this book. You *can* skip eating every now and then. You can look better and feel better and have the energy to do all the things you want to do—consciously, deliberately, freely.

FOOD ON THE BRAIN

Fasting makes you sharper. Well, of course it does. Think about what happens to animals when they don't eat: they become fully attuned to their environment so they can find food. That's another universal, fundamental evolutionary pressure, one that very much shaped what *Homo sapiens* is today.

As an illustration, I'll tell you a story an old friend of mine, a guy named Chris. He served in the army doing Special Forces–type long-range patrols in hostile territory. During training, his small team had to make their way across rough terrain wearing heavy backpacks, going for two or three days without any food. The point was to show them that they could do the seemingly impossible—schlep eighty-pound backpacks up mountains—while fasting. The training was intended to make the team feel as though they were starving and learn that the feeling wasn't true. To show the team how fasting sharpened their senses, the folks in charge of the training would hang a cheeseburger high up in a tree at their destination.

Chris told me he could smell that cheeseburger from two miles away. Don't believe it? Neither did I at first, but he swore it was true, and he's an honest guy. "Absolutely, one hundred percent of us could smell the cheeseburger," he said. "They didn't tell us they were going to put the cheeseburger there. We just smelled it. We knew it was there, and we were drawn to it."

That's the remarkable power of your body and your brain working in unison. When you skip eating for a whole twenty-four hours, your senses sharpen, and your focus increases. The less toxic material you have in your bloodstream and lymphatic system, the higher your ability to reason. This is because the tremendous amount of energy that your internal organs normally require for digestion is now being shunted to the brain. Once toxins have been eliminated, the brain begins receiving healthy, toxin-free blood, allowing it to use its resources more efficiently. Your capacity to focus on anything you want to increases as well, because your brain is no longer distracted by food. You can focus on your work, you can focus on how you feel, you can focus on your meditation—you can focus on whatever you want. Intricate problems that once stymied you may seem easy to resolve.

Many people report that fasting provides them insights into themselves like they've never felt before. On a long fast, the feelings of emotional stability and euphoria can be life changing. Why do you think every great religious practice involves periods of fasting? Why do unrelated cultures all around the world link fasting with spiritual enlightenment? Because when you sharpen your brain, you sharpen all of your abilities.

Now, it's important to manage your expectations. The first time you fast, your brain isn't going to be all that concerned with a higher state of enlightenment. If things were that easy, humans would never have stopped fasting. Instead, you're going have to train yourself not to think about cookies or whatever your craving happens to be. Keep in mind that every thought takes energy. It takes electrons. In the same way that every app you run on your phone sucks battery power, every thought in your head sucks *brainpower*.

On a daily basis, studies show that about 15 percent of your thoughts are some iteration of "What's for dinner? Do I need food right now?"[8] If you're on a diet, that number may be closer to 50 percent. Those food fixations are evolutionary relics that no longer serve a useful purpose, like your wisdom teeth or your appendix. (Actually, the appendix may serve a function in maintaining the vigor of your microbiome,[9] so your cravings are less useful than your appendix!) By kicking up your metabolism and powering up your neurons with ketones, intermittent fasting teaches the brain not to waste time on obsessive food thoughts.

After you've done some of the basic fasting using the techniques laid out in this book, I guarantee that the amount of time you spend thinking about food will decrease. And if you also cut down on the foods that cause inflammation, you may find it remarkable how quickly you can shut down those thoughts entirely. There's an old myth that humans use only 10 percent of their brains (totally untrue), which has inspired many fanciful stories about the astonishing things we could do if only we could tap into the full power of the modern, evolved brain. Well, here's something that's not myth at all but real and testable. You can cut down on food-related thinking and free up more time and energy in your brain for everything else—just through intermittent fasting.

Speaking of thinking, there are two primary types of cells in the brain, and they both influence our relationship with food and hunger. One is your neurons, the brain's rock stars; everyone knows about those. But there are also the glial cells, or just glia, which are a lot less famous even though they are just as abundant in the brain: you have about 100 billion of each. The glia provide structural support, insulation, management, and nutrition for the neurons. Significantly, they also function as the brain's immune system. The glia are the pruners and maintainers of the brain. When your glia get disturbed, that's when inflammation in the brain happens. Disturbed glia can trigger pain and stimulate overeating.[10]

That's not something you want.

Neurons and glia can both use glucose or fat for fuel, but they have radically different tastes. Glia run best when you have some glucose in your body for them to use, and they get stressed when blood sugar falls too low. Neurons run best when you have ketones from fat they can use as fuel, but they're happy to use sugar as a backup. In nature, if you're fasting, you have high ketones and happy neurons, and you feel great. If you're eating anything with carbs, you have less-energetic neurons but good brain maintenance by happy glia. Which is better?

Remember that neurons are extremely energy hungry; they need lots of chemical fuel so you can think at your full capacity. If you're really, truly hungry, your blood sugar's low, and you're not in ketosis. Here's what happens: you can't think clearly. Your reaction time is delayed, and you feel slow because your neurons aren't able to get enough raw material to make electricity. But if your brain and body are running on ketones instead of glucose, something remarkable happens: the ketones have an inflammation-calming effect on the glia, because ketones are anti-inflammatory. Fasting gives you those ketones, which calms the glia, which improves the function of your neurons, which makes your thinking sharper.

At least, that's the goal. If you're doing a multiday fast and your body needs glucose for high-priority functions such as brainpower, you will enter a state called *gluconeogenesis*. Some proponents of the paleo diet and the dirty keto diet fetishize gluconeogenesis. The idea is that once you enter this state, your body will make all the carbohydrates you need from the proteins in your body. Technically, it is true: if you're starving or on a really long fast, you can lose muscle, because your body will break down protein from your muscles to make carbohydrates. The problem is that turning protein into sugar is biologically very expensive. It also leaves all sorts of waste products in the body, including ammonia. Those waste products lead to inflammation, which in turn leads to cravings and the muffin top.

The dirty keto folks have a whole theory of why this is a good thing. And they're right that brief periods of protein deprivation help promote autophagy, but you don't need too much of a good thing. When you endlessly combine fasting and keto, you become metabolically inflexible because your cells don't handle carbohydrates well. You're better off to fast sometimes, be in ketosis sometimes (fasting from carbs), and be in carbohydrate-burning mode sometimes.

What you want to do is turn on that gluconeogenesis as fast as you can and get into ketosis as fast as you can. That is the goal of intermittent fasting, and Bulletproof Intermittent Fasting is designed to help get you there. When you burn ketones, you enable your glial cells to go efficiently about their brain maintenance and anti-inflammatory tasks—the tasks that evolution shaped them to do.

A TUNE-UP FOR YOUR MEMORY MACHINE

Intermittent fasting is crucial not just for your in-the-moment mental clarity but also for the long-term well-being of your brain. It's extremely difficult to gather clean clinical data on the effects of intermittent fasting on human brain health; such studies take a long time and require separating the effects of eating habits from all the other things people do. But recently there has been a lot of highly encouraging evidence from lab animal experiments.

In study after study with rodents, intermittent fasting has been shown to increase memory, learning, and neurogenesis—the generation of neural cells. A team at the National University of Singapore reported in 2019 that intermittent fasting particularly leads to the growth of new neurons in the hippocampus, a part of the brain associated with learning and the conversion of short-term recall to long-term memory.[11] Mark Mattson, the neuroscientist at Johns Hopkins University, has noted that fasting and exercise seem to boost a protein called brain-derived neurotrophic factor, or BDNF, which increases the number of energy-generating mitochondria in the hippocampus and also promotes neurogenesis.[12] Intriguingly, Mattson and his colleagues have found that fasting elevates levels of another protein, SIRT3 (Sirtuin 3), which causes the mitochondria in the hippocampus to operate more efficiently.[13] Sure enough, rats that undergo intermittent fasting perform better on learning and memory tasks.

Do these results apply to humans? I believe so. When I measured my hippocampal volume using a functional magnetic resonance imaging, or fMRI, machine, I was in the 87th percentile for my age. Given that your hippocampus shrinks over time, this is evidence that mine isn't shrinking or has at least grown back. Since I had chemically induced brain damage from toxic mold in my twenties, the odds are that mine has grown back. I'll take that!

If things go wrong in the brain, fasting seems to help there as well. Our friend Mattson and his colleagues ran yet another rodent study and found that fasting leads to faster recovery from stroke, apparently by taming inflammation in the brain and by speeding the repair of injured neurons.[14]

The jury is still out about to what extent fasting can protect against neurodegenerative disorders such as Alzheimer's and Parkinson's diseases, although a 2018 rodent study out of South Korea reported promising findings.[15] One possible link is that ketones, unlike glucose, do not contribute to the buildup of destructive plaques in the brain. Valter Longo, a gerontologist at the University of Southern California, is filling in more pieces of the puzzle. His research has shown that fasting decreases the biochemical markers for diabetes (an Alzheimer's risk factor), as well as cardiovascular disease and cancer. He concludes that fasting reprograms the brain's metabolism and helps clear out malfunctioning cells, including the self-destructive immune cells that cause multiple sclerosis.[16] High levels of BDNF are associated with a lower risk of developing Parkinson's, Alzheimer's, Huntington's, and multiple sclerosis. And by suppressing inflammation in the brain, fasting also seems to improve blood circulation, which in turn helps preserve cognitive health.

This long list of health benefits may seem hard to believe. How can fasting do so many good things for you? The answer is simple: your body is already packed full of repair and rejuvenation mechanisms. Thousands of years—no, millions of years—no, *billions* of years of evolution have shaped them inside of us. Your ancestors have run the gauntlet of death and extinction. You and I are the survivors of an inconceivably brutal winnowing process. We wouldn't be here if we didn't have all of those health-preserving cells and molecules.

All that fasting does is remove the dietary impediments we put in our own way and allows us to take maximal advantage of the gifts evolution has given us. Fasting puts us in control of a 4-billion-year-old evolutionary process.

In many ways, the most important way fasting puts you in control of your brain is that *it makes you feel better about yourself.* By associating food with certain times of the day, family gatherings, and emotional comforting (why do you think we call it "comfort food"?), we give it overwhelming power over us. In the process, we turn a blind eye to the foods we're eating—and the ways we're eating—that do the opposite of making us feel comforted or nurtured. A food hangover is a very real thing. It is the price we pay for indulging in certain low-quality, inflammatory, toxin-laced foods just because we've been conditioned to crave them or to derive short-term comfort from them.

Try this experiment in food awareness: For one single day, pay close attention to how your body feels after each meal. Really pay attention. Are you sluggish after eating a certain food? Revved up? Do you have minor abdominal discomfort? Or worse, *major* abdominal discomfort? As you go through this experiment, pay close attention to mood swings and anxiety—sensations not often associated with food but just as common. Think about how your brain and body are responding.

Through most of the history of our species, it was unusual to encounter sugar-rich foods that would deliver rapid spikes of calories. Many of the ingredients of the modern diet have been cultivated by humans for only a couple hundred years or less—far too little time for our bodies to have adapted to them. Modern wheat is full of starch. Modern fruit is a sweet piece of candy compared to wild sour apples. Modern corn, bursting with sugar, didn't exist in much of the world until recently. And canola oil was known as "rapeseed oil" and considered inedible until it was put through an elaborate industrial detoxification process. That doesn't necessarily mean that modern fruits, vegetables, or grains are bad, exactly, but research shows that most of them contain more sugar than is ideal, and some of them (such as corn, soy, and wheat) really do harm your gut bacteria or your metabolism. Intermittent fasting helps reduce the potential for that harm, regardless of what you're eating.

The inflammation that comes with eating manufactured foods also plays an important role in how our brain perceives emotional health. A glass of reconstituted orange juice is sugar water—nutritious sugar water, but sugar water nonetheless—that elevates your blood sugar in a hurry and brings you right back down in a hurry. Feelings of anger and increased hunger often follow. It goes without saying that sugar-sweetened soda does the same thing, just without the nutrition. But did you know that diet sodas can lead to feelings of depression? Modern artificial sweeteners mimic the taste of sugar so well that the receptors in your stomach have trouble distinguishing between real soda and diet soda, so they release insulin just the same.

So-called light salad dressing follows the same path, eschewing sugars and high-fructose corn syrup but using aspartame, an artificial sweetener linked to depression. Ketchup is loaded with sugar. Pasta and white bread are often made of highly processed white flour that quickly turns to blood sugar as you eat, resulting in energy spikes, depression, and anxiousness. Eating fried foods, pizza dough, cakes, cookies, and even crackers can lead to feelings of depression, as can eating candy, pastries, processed meat, and refined cereals. They are all out of sync with our dietary evolution. The more you practice fasting, the less you're tempted by these low-quality offerings from Big Food.

In addition to its cellular repair mechanisms, your brain also contains higher-level emotional repair mechanisms that are just waiting to be activated. After a period of fasting, the brain instructs the adrenal glands—two small triangular glands located in your lower back atop the kidneys—to release catecholamines. These chemicals are neurotransmitters, molecules that trigger focused neuronal responses. Back when our ancestors were mostly hunting for a living and often going days without eating, catecholamines served a vital survival function: they helped keep the hunter optimistic and prepared for the exertion of the pursuit. Catecholamines include several famous mood-altering and energy-boosting chemicals, including adrenaline, norepinephrine, cortisol, and dopamine. You may recognize these as the chemicals, or the chemical targets, that doctors often prescribe to battle depression and stress. Your body also uses them to stabilize your blood sugar should it fall too low during a fast.

How wonderful is it that your body produces these mood elevators naturally during fasting? This is the "go mode" I felt at the end of my vision quest (more about that soon). The same feelings of happiness and well-being are available to everyone, anytime, without pharmaceutical assistance.

Food is built into your evolutionary history. Taking control of your food consumption can be the key to your future happiness.

5

FAST FOR BETTER SLEEP; SLEEP FOR A BETTER FAST

At last I was heading into the solitary adventure I had yearned for from the start. Delilah drove me to a new trailhead and gave me directions to find First Woman cave, located about a half mile down a canyon.

The site was sacred, she warned me in stern tones, and had been used ceremonially for ten thousand years. It is called First Woman based on the mythology of the Yavapai tribe of Arizona. They believe that they are all descended from a woman named Kamalapukwia, whose offspring emerged from that cave in the Yavapai equivalent of the Adam and Eve myth. The cave also earned its name because its opening is shaped like a giant vagina. The resemblance was hard to miss as we were driving up. (Note: This is not a cave for tourism. I am being intentionally vague about some details to protect its rightful use by those with permission to be there. You will not find it online.)

It was my second time getting settled in a cave for my vision quest but the first time that it felt real. It was October, when the Sonoran Desert is still hot during the daytime but chilly at night. I was glad for my sleeping bag. The weather reminded me of autumn days when

I was growing up in New Mexico, where you knew you would either sweat or freeze. On the first day, when I ventured out of First Woman cave and into the livid sun, I took off my shirt, knowing that no one would see the stretch marks I was still ashamed of—scars from my hard-won battle with obesity.

Two days into my vision quest and two days into my very first long fast, I hiked a mile carrying a backpack. For newbies like me, the second day of a fast is when you feel the most hunger. I was getting that. The second day is also a time when exhilaration can kick in. I was getting that, too. Thank you, catecholamines!

I was becoming attuned to all of the physical detail around me. It felt as though my eyes could focus on every speck of dust inside the cave, though at the same time I could feel that the air was full of dirt particles that were far too fine to see. I explored the cave as far in as it went, pondering where among the endless uneven surfaces I should set up camp. It was a dry sandstone cave about thirty feet deep and twelve feet wide, with a roof low enough that I could touch it in most spots. The history all around me was palpable. How many tens of thousands of fires had built up the thick soot on the roof of the cave? Who had been here, and had their thoughts been anything like mine? Eventually my mind settled and I made my little camp on a nice, flat ledge halfway into the cave—a piece of the roof that had probably fallen down thousands of years before. I laid out my water and sleeping bag and ventured out to gather some sticks to make a fire.

After that, there was nothing else to do except wonder if a scorpion, rattlesnake, or some large predator would visit. I was alone—truly alone—in a cave, cut off from human support and sustenance. The dancing shadows from my fire had a hallucinogenic quality, and I was already in a hungry, meditative state. I thought about all the other people who must have looked at similar shadows flickering on the same wall in a cave that's been used for ceremonies for ten thousand years. From there my mind wandered all over the place, including into the forbidding corners of fear and loneliness.

It felt like an impossible task in the utter darkness of that lonely cave, but I tried to get some rest. I was trying to listen to the rhythms of my body and trying to feel liberated from food and companionship. My imagination kept conjuring up visions of a very large snake slithering up to eat me. Eventually, though, sleep won out and my consciousness slipped away.

SLEEP CLEAN; GET CLEAN WHILE YOU SLEEP

Getting a good night's sleep is one of the most powerful ways you can enhance the impact of your fast. From a simple bookkeeping point of view, the connection between the two is obvious: while you're sleeping you aren't eating, so sleeping makes it a hell of a lot easier to get through the hours of a 16:8 fast. The connection goes way beyond that, though. Sleeping, like fasting, influences cellular and biochemical processes throughout the body. Combine intermittent fasting with healthy sleep patterns (what researchers call "good sleep hygiene"), and the results are synergistic.

You can easily understand how vital sleep is, even if you know nothing about what it does for you. On average we spend a full one-third of our lives unconscious, immobilized, and unresponsive to sights and sounds. That's fine for modern people snoozing away in our cozy bedrooms, but think what all of those sleeping hours meant for our ancestors: they spent one-third of their time utterly defenseless against attack. Sleep seems like a terrible survival strategy, something that would have quickly been weeded out by evolution, yet every person does it. Every animal alive sleeps, and as near as scientists can tell,[1] that's the way things have been since animals first appeared on Earth more than 500 million years ago, during the Ediacaran period.[2] Evolution is ruthlessly efficient. If sleep is ubiquitous, that means it must be essential to life—more important, even, than being able to run away from a predator that wants to eat you. We have to treat it with respect.

Have you ever gone a full day or more without sleep and felt as though you were going to drop dead? Death by sleep deprivation is a real thing. In a famous 1989 study,[3] researchers at the University of Chicago actually observed it happen to a group of lab rats. (It would be completely unethical to run the equivalent experiment on humans, but there's every reason to think that the danger is equally real for us.) Humans will die from lack of sleep long before they die from lack of food, yet most people would instinctively choose to be tired instead of hungry.

Conversely, you know how sharp and focused you feel after a particularly restful sleep? It seems as though every day there's another study backing up that feeling and scientifically documenting the benefits of a good night's sleep. The nightly hours of inactivity provide an opportunity to regenerate, both mentally and physically. This is the time when your subconscious mind solves problems and your muscles rest and grow stronger through increased protein production. During sleep, inflammation in the brain is flushed away by the recently discovered glymphatic system,[4] in which glial cells open up little garbage chutes to remove cellular waste from the cerebrospinal fluid. The cleansing action of the glymphatic system appears to reduce the risk of Alzheimer's disease and other brain disorders; it may slow overall aging of the brain as well. Sleeping six and a half to eight hours each night appears to reduce the risk of heart attack by staving off high blood pressure. There's also evidence that getting a good night's sleep reduces your risk of developing cancer via multiple mechanisms, including higher melatonin levels, reduced inflammation, and cellular repair as protein-digesting enzymes get to work while you slumber.

Yet 35 percent of Americans report that they regularly get fewer than seven hours of sleep a night, according to statistics collected by the Centers for Disease Control and Prevention (CDC).[5] There's a good chance that you're one of them, and there's a 100 percent chance that the CDC didn't ask whether people get *good* sleep even if they sleep more than seven hours. So before we even get into the potent connections between sleep and fasting, consider the importance of sleep itself:

- Sleep reduces stress.

- Sleep reduces inflammation.

- Sleep speeds healing.

- Sleep enhances cognitive function and memory, making you sharp and alert.

- Sleep enhances your sex drive.

- And yes, sleep helps you lose weight.

Unless you're sleeping in a jungle where a predator might attack you at any moment under the cover of darkness, there's no downside to getting a good night's sleep. Fasting can help you do just that.

Strictly speaking, the period of time you spend sleeping is time spent fasting. That's how the meal of breakfast gets its name: literally "break-fast." If you choose to skip breakfast and go a few more hours without sleeping, you have now begun intermittent fasting. Keep fasting just a few hours past the time when you wake up, and your body significantly reduces the secretion of insulin while it increases secretion of human growth hormone, or HGH. This is important, because HGH aids in cellular repair, encourages fat burning, and assists in the development of lean muscle mass.

To maximize the benefits of this process, you should wait at least six hours after rising before you eat your first meal. Your sleep cycle also helps set the time when you should finish eating for the day. If you eat late in the evening, particularly close to bedtime, your body will still be actively engaged in the digestion process when you lie down for the night. All that food in your gut is a signal to your circadian timing system that it must be near daytime still, because humans aren't nocturnal! Devoting all of that metabolic energy to digestion can make it more difficult for you to fall asleep. Your blood glucose and insulin levels also stay elevated for a longer time after an evening meal than when you eat during the day, which can lead to an elevated risk of glucose intolerance, type 2 diabetes, and high blood pressure. For the past several years, I've used continuous blood glucose monitoring designed for diabetics, and I've consistently noticed that a late dinner causes me to have higher blood sugar levels the next day, even during an intermittent fast. Skip the late dinners!

After you fall asleep, those elevated blood sugar and insulin levels can also cause you to awaken frequently, because your body is still engaged in digestion. You might not notice these times of wakefulness during the night, while you're in that half-asleep/half-awake fog. What you will notice is that you don't feel properly sharp and focused when you wake up for real in the morning. A simple way to find out about your sleep quality is to buy one of the many good commercial sleep-tracking devices. At the time of publication, the best device is the Oura ring, which is used by professional athletes such as NBA players to track their sleep, and the best phone-only sleep tracker is the SleepSpace app. They will pinpoint how many times you wake up during the night. The results might make you think twice about late-night snacking. Good sleep hygiene and good fasting habits go hand in hand.

Ideally, you should always leave *at least* three hours between your meal and the time you go to sleep. Ruth Patterson and Dorothy Sears, health researchers at the University of California San Diego, recently conducted a thorough review of the literature on the link between eating and sleeping.[6] They concluded that each three-hour increase in the gap between the last meal and bedtime significantly reduces the odds of elevated blood sugar levels and elevated levels of C-reactive protein, an indicator of inflammation. Other studies show that working the night shift triggers many of the same negative biological responses as eating right before sleep and that fasting can offset those issues.

Again, good sleep hygiene and good fasting habits go hand in hand. As for why they do—well, that's a whole fascinating story in itself.

YOUR INNER CLOCK

Our bodies are guided by an internal clock known as the circadian rhythm. It dictates when we fall asleep and how we wake up. It also directs when cells should activate different energy-producing chemical pathways, such as burning fats instead of sugars while we're asleep. Eating too close to bedtime brings on metabolic dysfunction because it conflicts with your natural circadian rhythm. The culprit isn't just the food you're eating, then, but your body itself—specifically, a tiny region of the brain called the suprachiasmatic nucleus, located just behind the eyes. The suprachiasmatic nucleus is the master time-keeper, sending out chemical signals that instruct us when to sleep and when to awaken.

Broadly speaking, the circadian rhythm evolved to synchronize the sleep-wake cycle with the rising and setting of the sun. The existence of biological rhythms as an internal clock, and not just a response to day and night, was first noted in 640 BCE by the Greek poet Archilochus of Paros, who wrote that we need to "recognize which rhythms govern man." (Archilochus is also the author of the insightful aphorism "The fox knows many things, the hedgehog one big thing." There's great value in being a hedgehog who pays attention to foundational truths, rather than a fox who gets distracted by many little details.)

From there it took an astonishingly long time to learn more about the clock inside us. The French astronomer Jean-Jacques d'Ortous de Mairan deduced the existence of a regular biological rhythm in plants in 1729, more than two millennia after Archilochus. The discovery of equivalent rhythms in animals didn't happen until early in the twentieth century. Progress was so slow that the biologists Jeffrey C. Hall, Michael Rosbash, and Michael W. Young won a Nobel Prize in Physiology or Medicine "for their discoveries of molecular mechanisms controlling the circadian rhythm"—in 2017![7]

We now know that the circadian clock regulates a wide variety of metabolic processes so that they recur every day at the optimal time for the functioning and survival of the organism. Daylight helps reset this rhythm, but it keeps on ticking inside us even if we don't see sunrise and sunset. Unfortunately, the modern lifestyle doesn't always align with that ticking, in much the same way that today's scheduled eating patterns run counter to the way our species evolved. Our master clock is easily influenced by outside stimuli, including social events, screen time, and that late-night snack you popped into your mouth ten minutes before going to bed.

Sleep researchers sometimes call these stimuli *zeitgebers*, which is not as rude as it sounds; it means "time givers" in German. Zeitgebers can prompt your liver, muscle, and fatty tissue to be active at times when they should be shutting down for the night. The brain, meanwhile, can get confused when this occurs, attempting to prepare the body for bed based on time of day and your normal sleep pattern, even as specific organs and tissues are kicking into a high state of action. The resulting disruption of the circadian rhythm triggers inflammation and altered immune responses; those changes, in turn, can further mess with the rhythm, leading to a vicious cycle.

One potential result, according to a 2017 study out of the University of Sydney in Australia, is a cascade of inflammatory-related respiratory diseases, including chronic obstructive pulmonary disease, allergic rhinitis, and asthma.[8] Or, more succinctly, "trouble."

But even as your binge watching and Instagram swiping and ill-timed snacking are insulting your body with zeitgebers, placing a time restriction on when you eat can switch the body into a more consistent sleep routine. Establishing a routine makes it easier to fall asleep and allows you to wake up naturally without the jarring shriek of an alarm. And as with the natural mood enhancement provided by the body's release of endorphins during a fast, you don't have to stick any medications into your body. You don't need sleeping pills or other pharmacological assistance to fall into a deep natural sleep. You merely need to get your circadian rhythms into working order.

I know. That word, *merely*, may seem to downplay the challenge. How are you going to go without your Netflix and social media and all of your comfort food? Remember, *going without* does not mean *going without everything*. Remember, too, that I have a whole set of biohacks to share with you, ways that emphasize your sense of control and steer you away from suffering. You can have your cake and eat it, too, if you know how your body works and when to eat it!

SNOOZE YOUR WAY INTO AN EASY FAST

Intermittent fasting is a biohack that will help you with sleeping. Restful sleeping is a biohack that will help you with fasting. How cool is that?

It's common for people on their second night of fasting (or longer) to need less sleep. In fact, people typically find they need an hour less sleep each night during a multiday fast, while they're intermittent fasting, or even while they're just eating less inflammatory food. Alertness and the production of neurochemicals that stimulate wakefulness in the brain increase during daytime periods of fasting, but the levels of those chemicals tend to decrease at night, which supports deep sleep. The way a healthy sleep curve works is that during the first half of the night, you get your deep sleep. During the second half, you get your rapid eye movement, or REM, sleep, when you do your intense dreaming. If you wake up an hour earlier during your fast, you're going to get less REM; if you go to bed an hour later, you're going to get less deep sleep. Either way, you are going to wake up feeling more refreshed than before you started fasting.

Think of fasting as a gift. That hour not spent sleeping is a bonus time in your day to read, write, meditate, enjoy your friends and family, and generally just be good to yourself. An hour a day for a year works out to fifteen full twenty-four-hour days saved, or about six weeks of working eight hours a day. Is eating a late dinner really worth throwing that gift of time away?

Establishing an eating window will do a lot to help you reap these benefits. That's easier than it sounds, because society already runs on regular mealtimes. That gives you a ready structure to start with. Now make it your own. My personal eating window is between noon and 6:00 p.m. in winter, when it gets dark early, and from 2:00 to as late as 8:00 p.m. in summer. Earlier is better. Nothing after dark is ideal. Or you might say, "I'm going to eat only between 10:00 a.m. and 2:00 p.m." if a schedule like that works for your life. The key is to pick a schedule that makes sense to you and that you can sustain comfortably. You may find that late business dinners get in the way. In those situations, I usually eat my real dinner on time, then go to the business dinner and pick at a salad to make other people feel better about their late dinner.

Having a window doesn't mean you should eat anything you want during those six or eight hours of consumption. This isn't a dirty keto diet or the Coke and Doritos diet—not even the plant-based Coke and Doritos diet. You'll be much happier if you eat simple, healthy meals. But even if you do follow the Coke and Doritos diet, eating them in moderation and not putting any food into your mouth three hours before bedtime will still result in weight loss and better sleep.

The most workable intermittent fasting schedule for all but the most extreme is to skip breakfast, then eat lunch and dinner. It seems extravagant to call such a straightforward guideline a "biohack," but that's really what it is. Create an eating rhythm that supports your sleep rhythm and the circadian rhythm that underpins all of it. Don't consume your nightly meal too late. The breakfast-skipping approach to fasting is very pragmatic. The strongest possible circadian-supporting schedule is to plan your eating window in the morning—breakfast and lunch, then no dinner—but few people can stick to it because it's not worth the social awkwardness that comes from skipping dinners.

For some people, especially those like me who have a hard time sleeping or going to bed on time, the impact of fasting is much more pronounced if you strictly follow the "no food after dark" rules. For people who suffer from moderate to severe sleep apnea, consuming calories close to bedtime can increase the number of sleep disturbances (caused by lack of oxygen to the brain due to throat closure) that happen during the night and can contribute to a lack of deep, restful sleep. On the other hand, going without dinner entirely is tough for beginning fasters.

Here's a tip to help you fall asleep more quickly while not feeling hungry when you go to bed: when you sit down for dinner, indulge in some white rice and a little sweet potato. You may say it sounds as though I'm contradicting myself: I'm suggesting you eat carbs, and carbs are the enemy of ketosis. Think of this as fine tuning, keeping some flexibility in your fast. Don't overindulge, but a little dose of carbs at dinner can be really helpful in reducing physical anxiety. Carbs produce serotonin, a neurotransmitter (brain-signaling chemical) known to help us fall asleep. By eating a dinner including a tiny bit of carbs three to four hours before bedtime, you set yourself up for a deeper, more restful night of sleep.

So long as it's just a modest bite or two of carbs, you can eat it and stay in ketosis if you have MCT oil with it. You might even enjoy a small dessert containing a few grams of sugar or, ideally, a little bit of raw honey once or twice a week. This can take you out of ketosis for a little while, but you will go right back after a short fast. The reason I recommend raw honey is that it raises the level of glycogen in the liver. Liver glycogen preferentially feeds the brain. And as much as your muscles regenerate and recuperate during a good night's sleep, it's your brain that benefits the most from that period of rest. It needs a full energy supply to do its cleansing and regeneration. Good sleep, good eating, and good brain health all go hand in hand.

There is one important disclaimer: it's entirely possible that you will get into a state where you wake up in the middle of the night while fasting, especially when you first start out. Don't despair; you're not doing anything wrong. You're still on the path to better sleep and improved cognitive function. What you're experiencing is the effect of cortisol, a hormone that acts like an alarm signal in the body. It's sending a message that you should have a few carbs or skip a day or two of intermittent fasting.

People often talk about cortisol as if it's the enemy. Health reporters typically describe it as the hormone that's related to too much stress, coffee consumption, sitting, and negative emotion in our lives. Some people also connect high cortisol levels with adrenal fatigue, which is a real problem. (I can attest to that, because I've had it before; adrenal fatigue can cause lethargy, aches, disrupted sleep, and digestive problems.) But as with all the chemicals your body makes, cortisol has a damn good reason for being there. It turns out that having low cortisol is much worse than having high cortisol. If you don't have enough cortisol, your body's ability to make energy, as well as to control inflammation—and even to maintain the baseline blood pressure we need to think—is impaired. When your metabolism is trained to fast, your cells switch easily between burning glucose and burning ketones, you have more energy, and your cortisol levels will likely resolve to become like Goldilocks's favorite chair: not too big, not too small, just right!

If fasting makes your body believe it's running out of energy—particularly glucose—your body will pump out cortisol as a quick fix because cortisol immediately raises blood sugar, which is a mechanism meant to keep you alive. This is similar to the fight-or-flight response that fills you with energy if you feel that you're in danger. The first thing the brain does is declare an emergency. It triggers a rapid secretion of cortisol and adrenaline to create blood sugar. Your whole body goes into a state of high alert. That's why I call nighttime cortisol production a chemical alarm signal.

When you start fasting, this emergency process can kick in at a particularly inconvenient moment, around three o'clock in the morning. To the brain, this time coincides with a critical part of the sleep cycle when it needs access to a lot of energy so it can wash itself free of toxins. This process, called glymphatic circulation, is very important for consolidating memories and putting them into your long-term recall. As part of your middle-of-the-night brain wash, your neurons pump out their water, getting rid of the toxic proteins that built up during the day. The brain then replenishes itself with fresh, clean cerebral spinal fluid so you can wake up and feel good the next day.

This is a beautiful thing if the process unfolds the way it's supposed to. But beginning fasters—or unending keto cultists—can get an unwelcome surprise if the fight-or-flight, where's-my-energy response kicks in during the night. By releasing cortisol and adrenaline, the brain rapidly gets the energy it needs for glymphatic circulation. Your individual neurons are happy and clean. However, the whole you—the person reading this book—won't be so happy. The 3:00 a.m. freak-out includes racing thoughts and an inability to go back to sleep. If this happens to you, try eating a little raw honey before bed. It's an easy fix to keep you going until your body adapts to fasting. A little bit of sweetness will keep your brain content and will keep you content, too. If carbs don't work for you, even a little MCT oil can help by increasing the level of circulating ketones, which provide alternate energy for your brain.

RESPECT THE RHYTHM OF LIFE

You've begun the process of taking control of your circadian rhythm, making it part of your program to own your biology. To keep going, you'll want to know even more about how your internal clock works. The circadian rhythm is responsible for much more than regulating sleep and wakefulness; it also promotes a healthy metabolism and immune system, which helps explain why good sleep is associated with such a vast range of positive health effects.

Your circadian rhythms exert a delicate, complex influence on all of the 30 trillion cells in your body. Its impact goes even deeper than that. Each active cell contains hundreds to thousands of mitochondria that drive your metabolism by extracting the chemical energy from the food you eat. Ideally, every single mitochondrion in your body knows when it's day and when it's night. And just as ideally, all of them act in unison, responding to the chemical signals of the circadian rhythm and mediating the way it is expressed in your changing mood, energy levels, and activity levels over the course of the day.

But this delicate dance can fall apart in response to sensory signals that clash with the rhythm. The strongest signal of all is the one that tells the brain whether it's day or night: light. Cells in your eyes continuously measure the color, strength, and angle of the light around you and shuttle that information to the suprachiasmatic nucleus, to other parts of the brain, and beyond. I'm not talking about the things you see. I'm talking about much more subtle observations, ones you don't consciously recognize even though they affect you to the core. Your circadian rhythm is constantly adjusting and resetting in response to nature's light cycles. When you surround yourself with artificial light—which hits you with unnatural colors at unnatural hours—your rhythm changes. Your mitochondria change. Your exquisitely evolved biochemical dance can stumble into metabolic dysfunction. And when that light tweaks the function of your mitochondria, your blood sugar level is impacted, too.

That's why I deliberately create an optimal sleep environment. I wear glasses that filter out junk light at night, and I dim the lights before bedtime as much as possible or use sleep-friendly light bulbs (more on this in a minute). I cover my windows with blackout curtains and make my bedroom into my own personal cave. Even if you're not ready to go quite that far, you should be mindful of your evening illumination. It's critically important that you turn down your lights at night, especially during fasting. If you don't, you will end up undoing a lot of your good work. Yes, you can go on a bright-light-at-night fast, too.

You should also reduce, if not cease altogether, looking at screens when it gets close to bedtime. No TV. No laptops. No phones. One hour before going to sleep is a good goal to aim for. Electronic screens emit a blue-enhanced light that resembles the rays of the midday sun. Finely tuned optical receptors in your eye are tricked into thinking it's still daytime. Those receptors trigger the secretion of hormones to keep you awake and suppress the levels of sleep-inducing melatonin. When you finally do fall asleep, the lingering effect of the blue-tinged screens means that your sleep won't be as deep or restful.

Paul Gringas at King's College London helped raised awareness of this issue back in 2015.[9] Since then, many electronics companies have added a darker, redder "night mode" to their phones. In 2008, I had a custom pair of glasses made to block the types of light that ruin sleep, and since then I have continued research, filed patents, and started a company called TrueDark that makes special light bulbs and eyeglasses to reduce your exposure to daylight-simulating rays at night. (You can do everything in this book without using my glasses, but they work, so I'm sharing them with you here.) The truth is that if you dim your lights, use the glasses, and heavily dim your screens, it's possible to use screens right up until bedtime. I do it a lot, then sleep like a baby, but you have to be militant about your light exposure.

Still, these hacks are no substitute for switching off entirely. That's because restricting the amount of time you spend in front of the TV or staring at your devices is also a great first step toward a dopamine fast. I'll tell you more about how to do that in chapter 10. The key idea here is to cut back not just on the bluish light but on the whole addictive pattern of looking at videos, texts, and social media all the time. This is another craving that you can master and one that will help you feel more alive.

What you really want to do is attend to all of the factors that affect your sleep hygiene so that you optimize the way that sleep and intermittent fasting support each other. It's harder to fast when you get a bad night's sleep. You can start working on your sleep even before you begin your first fast. If you're like most people, the time you fall asleep and the time you wake up are determined more by habit and obligations than by what your body wants or what's best for you. Work on developing a plan that allows for a consistent six and a half to eight hours of rest each night. Think about when you really want to go to bed and when you want to wake up. Then you can decide where to place your "sleep window"—the hours that you choose, for yourself, to be your period of restoration.

Two things that are going to tell your body that it is time to wake up and shut your sleep window: bright light (especially sunlight) and available calories. Experiment to determine if there are new times when you might want to begin and end your sleep. If those times don't line up with what your body is doing now, you can hack them with fasting and light.

HOW TO DO A CIRCADIAN RESET FAST

Another way to tap into evolutionary patterns of sleep and fasting to your benefit is what I call the *circadian reset fast*. You use it for a short period to rapidly change your sleep/wake cycle to better fit the life you want, to fix jet lag, or to deal with shift work.

I've been tracking my sleep for fourteen years. As an author and as someone who likes to dive deep into research, I find that there's an especially productive writing time that happens very late at night. It's quiet. It's a time when I can focus. And since nobody else in my home is awake then, it's a great period of alone time. As much as I enjoy those late hours, they come at a cost. In the morning, I still have to take the kids to school at the usual hour. Staying up until 2:00 a.m. and then waking up five hours later over and over wears me down. It would wear anyone down. After a while, that kind of schedule makes you feel like garbage in the morning, and you wonder whether the exhilaration of the late-night creative burst is really worth it.

So of course, I decided to search for a biohack that would help me sleep normally when I'm done writing a book like this one. (It is 3:00 a.m. as I type this; it's when I tap into my best writing mode.)

In order to hack sleep, you have to hack billion-year-old evolutionary mechanisms, ones that predate the origin of animals—even the origin of sleep itself. I'm talking about back when the most complex form of life on Earth was single-cell bacteria floating in the ocean. Peak nutrients were available at noon, when the sun was highest. The sun would come up, and those ancestral bacteria would float up from the cold depths of the ocean. They would reach the surface and get their first jolt of morning sunlight, which would be a reddish color—because, hey, that's what sunrise looks like when you're floating in a primordial ocean. And then they would start getting energy from the sun and begin feasting on whatever was in the water around them. That whole legacy still lives on inside of you. The daily cycle of light and nutrition is encoded into your cells, and it's persisted for eons because it's kept us in sync with our planet. By selectively *going without*—without food, artificial light, or electronic distractions—you can restore harmony with your ancient internal rhythm.

You're going to combine the timing of food and sleep to trick your brain into moving your sleep window. Think about the stimuli that affect your body clock. The first is light, including its color, intensity and angle. The second is calories, or rather calories consumed. You can tweak this if you know how to fast. If you believe you'll starve without three meals a day, your sleep window will remain frustratingly out of your control! There aren't yet any ironclad studies to back up my theory, but I estimate that light controls about 70 percent of the strength of your circadian rhythm, food about 20 percent. And room temperature is probably the other 10 percent. These are the variables we're going to work on hacking to reset our circadian rhythm. The formula I've come up with boils down to this:

- Wake at the new time, with or without an alarm.

- Turn on bright indoor lights (halogen are best), or go outside without sunglasses.

- Drink coffee (with butter and C8 MCT oil) and have at least 30 to 50 grams of protein within thirty minutes of waking.

- Eat lunch normally, including lots of fat and grass-fed protein.

- Fast from 2:00 p.m. onward.

- Dim the lights and/or put on TrueDark glasses two hours before bed.

- Repeat for a week, and do not eat dinner at all—you are looking at a "reverse intermittent fasting" schedule where you eat all your calories in a morning eating window.

This formula works astoundingly well. I reliably went to sleep at about 2:00 to 4:00 a.m. for most of the last fourteen years. I just don't get tired until then. Using the above techniques, I now get tired and go to sleep at 11:00 p.m. and wake without alarm clock six and a half to seven hours later. I wish I'd known about these sleep hacks when I had a day job!

On the other side of the coin, if you happen to be the rare person who goes to bed at 9:00 p.m. and wakes at 4:00 a.m. and you want to reset your clock, you can use the same basic techniques to shift your bedtime later.

- Eat dinner an hour after dark, including lots of protein and a few carbs.

- Keep bright lights on for an hour (or maybe two) after the sun goes down.

- Avoid caffeine at night.

- Sleep in a very dark room.

- Wake up as late as you can.

- After you wake up, use low lighting and/or wear TrueDark glasses for one to two hours.

- Do not drink coffee until two hours after you wake up.

- Do not eat food of any type in the morning; butter and C8 MCT oil in your coffee are okay if you're hungry.

- Eat a late lunch at 2:00 p.m., including lots of fat and grass-fed protein.

- Repeat for a week.

It is truly remarkable how combining fasting with light can recalibrate your body's internal clock.

BRINGING ORDER TO DISORDERED SLEEP

So far, we've been discussing what you could call universal sleep problems: difficulty falling asleep, restless sleep, difficulty waking up, not enough sleep—the kinds of problems virtually all of us have. Adjusting your sleep window and your eating window will improve all of these issues. But a huge number of people also suffer from more specific sleep disorders. Intermittent fasting and taking control of your sleep schedule can help here, too.

The best-known sleep disorder is snoring, or sleep apnea as more severe cases are called. Sleep surveys suggest that up to 7 percent of the population suffers from apnea.[10] For snoring (formally defined as the sound air makes as it flows over relaxed tissues in your throat, forcing them to vibrate) the numbers are drastically higher.

If you stop eating several hours before bedtime so that your body can complete the first parts of the digestive process, it will help with your overall quality of sleep and should help tame mild to moderate snoring as well. The problem is that many of us lead hectic lives and can't always follow ideal eating patterns.

Let's say you're with an important client in a distant city. Your business dinner runs late, so by the time you get back to your hotel and you're ready to hit the hay, it's been just an hour since you ate. You're aware that this isn't optimal and that your body is still busy turning that food into energy, keying up your metabolism at a time when your circadian rhythm wants to shut you down for the night. Still, you do your best. You don't turn on the TV. You close the blackout drapes to banish outside light from your temporary castle. Maybe you use something like the SleepSpace app on your phone as a white-noise machine to create a neutral-sounding environment and duplicate your at-home sleep experience.

But then you toss and turn all night. You wake up with dry mouth, which means that you've been sleeping with your mouth open. Clearly you were snoring. In the morning, as you sip your coffee and try to arouse your mental acuity, you find yourself mildly exhausted. What went wrong?

First, your stomach was still somewhat full at bedtime. A full belly means that your diaphragm has less room to expand and contract (or, as you would more commonly say, "to rise and fall"). Your internal organs were crammed tightly into your abdominal cavity, pressed against one another like commuters on a rush-hour subway. A full stomach presses upward on the diaphragm, which in turn puts pressure on your lungs, not allowing them to expand completely. There is some evidence that sleeping on your left side can reduce pressure on the stomach, which is a good habit when you go to sleep on a full stomach. The rest of the time, sleeping on your right side is better for your heart.

Second, there's a good chance that you ate something you're sensitive to—even if you didn't know it—which triggered acid reflux or even anxiety. Those foods can relax the valve separating the esophagus and stomach. Acidic foods irritate the throat lining, leading to acid reflux. This is the condition that occurs when foods enter the stomach and then travel backward up the esophagus into the airway. (*Flux* is the Latin word for "flowing," and *reflux* is a flow going in the wrong direction.) Acid reflux can be severe enough to cause postnasal drip, another leading cause of snoring. This is excess mucus buildup on the back of the nose and throat. Dairy products, wheat, and alcohol are common triggers of mucus formation, too.

A late meal leads to acid reflux, which leads to postnasal drip, all of which then leads to coughing, airway irritation, and inflammation. Coughing is another leading cause of snoring, so it all adds up. Bad food plus bad timing equals bad sleep.

You may think that you had no control over all the factors that led to your lousy night's sleep and groggy morning—but of course you did. Perhaps you could have set the time of the dinner. Definitely you had control over what you ordered (wine? carbs? cheese sticks?). And definitely—*definitely*—you had control over when you went to bed. In this case, it would have been a smart trade to go to bed a little later, sacrificing some of your night's sleep *length* in exchange for better sleep *quality*: less sleep overall, but higher quality sleep. It's a good trade. You could also have taken a sleep-inducing supplement, such as melatonin, magnesium, or 5-hydroxytryptophan (5-HTP, also known as oxitriptan), to help.

Managing a more serious problem such as chronic obstructive sleep apnea is more difficult. This potentially fatal sleep disruption occurs when the soft tissues in the throat relax completely, blocking your airway. Sufferers wake up dozens of times a night gasping or choking and typically snore loudly enough that their partners cannot sleep. Wall-rattling snoring is the opposite of sexy, and the inevitable requests that the snorer sleep in another room can put quite a strain on a relationship. Adding insult to injury, one of sleep apnea's primary side effects—in addition to high blood pressure and nighttime sweating—is loss of libido.

Fasting alone can't completely fix sleep apnea. If you suffer from apnea, you need to begin by doing a sleep study with a reputable lab and getting treatment with a bite guard that helps your jaw stay forward or perhaps a CPAP machine. But to the extent that fasting can lead to weight loss, it can be a significant help. The number one cause of sleep apnea is being overweight, perhaps because of fatty deposits that accumulate in the upper airways. A recent study at the Perelman School of Medicine at the University of Pennsylvania uncovered a related risk factor: people who have excess tongue fat suffer disproportionately from sleep apnea.[11] There's no way to do liposuction of the tongue, unfortunately. Some research suggests that dronabinol, a cannabinoid drug, taken before bedtime could help. What clearly does work, though, is losing weight. A 10 percent reduction in body weight is associated with a 20 percent decrease in apnea symptoms, researchers have found.[12] Fasting to the rescue again!

Restless legs syndrome is another common sleep disorder, even though it is much less widely discussed than apnea. Also known as Willis-Ekbom disease, restless legs syndrome affects some 5 percent of the general population and 10 percent of people over the age of sixty-five.[13] As the name suggests, this syndrome leads to uncontrollable leg movements. This occurs most often at night as a series of little muscle spasms and can significantly affect quality of rest. Many people aren't even aware that they have it; all they know is that they tend to have low-quality sleep and frequently wake up feeling tired.

Although the connection is not as definitive as it is with apnea, restless legs syndrome appears to correlate with obesity.[14] There's also some evidence that restless legs syndrome may be brought on by mild neurological inflammation and nervous system disruption by toxins, heavy metals, environmental mold, and eating foods to which one is allergic. If you have restless legs, there's an easy way to tell if toxins from your diet are causing it: run a fasting experiment. Fast for a day, and go to sleep. If your restless legs are magically cured, it's likely that something in your diet is causing them. I used to have restless legs intermittently and discovered that by removing foods I was sensitive to, such as those high in histamine, lectins, and particularly mold toxins, my restless legs went away. Fasting will tell you if your restless legs are due to a food issue or something else.

YOU *DON'T* NEED A DRINK

Speaking of toxins, any meaningful program to improve your quality of sleep and exert self-control over your diet has to deal with the toxin that so many of us knowingly and eagerly consume.

Alcohol is fun to drink, and it is absolutely, positively bad for you.

Even a glass of wine several nights a week will destroy your sleep quality. You will see this as soon as you buy a sleep-tracking ring or wrist monitor; it will be blindingly obvious, no matter how much you don't want it to be true. Dr. Daniel Amen, a well-known psychiatrist and brain-health expert, has published 3D scans of brains of people who drink one glass of wine several nights a week, showing obvious metabolic brain dysfunctions as a result.

That said, drinking alcohol is fun as long as you do it with your eyes open. If you're going to drink, drink the most expensive stuff: you'll get the most enjoyment, and you'll end up drinking less. Be aware that alcohol breaks your fast and that your blood sugar level will likely be less stable the following day. You will need the intermittent fast even more the next morning, but it will be harder than usual to do. We all have our indulgences, though, so feel free to consume alcohol in moderation. The goal here is not misery, nor is it asceticism.

Perhaps the most surprising dietary aspect of alcohol is that it triggers a stress response that causes the body to secrete protective molecules called heat shock proteins. If you want to impress your friends with an argument *for* drinking alcohol, here it is: alcohol causes a short-term increase in body temperature and raises your heat shock proteins. That's why snow rescue dogs used to carry a little cask of brandy on their collars—so that hypothermic people could get a quick burst of heat from drinking it. That effect may explain the positive correlation between light to moderate alcohol intake and the risk of cardiovascular mortality seen in the landmark Zutphen Study, which tracked the health of 1,373 men over a period of forty years.[15] Unfortunately, the downside is still higher than the upside, and you can protect your heart a lot more effectively simply by fasting. Sorry.

While you're fasting or just lowering inflammation, you can choose alcohols that are lower in toxins and lower in sugar. At daveasprey .com/alcohol there is a full-page alcohol road map to help you select the best alcohol for fasting or just staying alive longer. It will help you drink intelligently. Distilled beverages without additives—vodka, tequila, and whiskey—are the best by far. Dry white French wine is your next best bet. After that, red wine. The worst of all is beer.

I get it: alcohol brings people a lot of pleasure, and it's deeply embedded in our social traditions. I just see an awful lot of people drinking in ways that don't take into account the true effects of alcohol. In particular, keep in mind this crucial fact: *alcohol is not a sleep aid*.

Contrary to the old tradition of having a "nightcap," drinking alcohol in the evening actually increases sleep interruption. True, it helps you fall asleep faster, but the type of sleep one experiences after that nightcap is not the deep, rapid eye movement (REM) sleep that promotes dreams and restores our brains. Then, when the alcohol wears off in the middle of the night, it ends up disrupting your sleep cycle. Like eating a large meal too close to bedtime, drinking alcohol causes sleep disruptions as the soft tissue of the throat becomes relaxed and possibly even completely closed. Drinking alcohol too close to bedtime can lead to sleepwalking, sleep talking, and memory problems.

There are no hard-and-fast rules about drinking while intermittent fasting, but always make sure to fill your stomach first. In other words, don't drink your calories. Also, since alcohol and fasting both place greater fluid needs on the body, make sure to drink plenty of water throughout both the fasting and nonfasting portions of your day. It's all about balance. If you're going to make fasting part of your lifestyle, avoid being extreme. Drink and eat in moderation, and don't beat yourself up if you're not perfect.

It's worth mentioning that *alcohol is not a sex aid, either.* If you want a better sex life, you're much more likely to get it by improving the quality of your sleep and embracing intermittent fasting. In a long-term study on fasting at the Pennington Biomedical Research Center in Baton Rouge, Louisiana, 218 people of a healthy weight (not obese or suffering from an eating disorder) agreed to reduce their caloric intake by 25 percent over a period of two years. Those who chose fasting as their means of caloric reduction reported a typical weight loss of about 16.5 pounds. In addition, the subjects said they slept better, felt happier, and enjoyed a better sex life.[16]

The key here is food choice while fasting. If you eat a diet high in protein and healthy fat during times of nonfasting, your sex drive will likely increase. If your diet has a deficit of healthy protein and fats—or if it is, in fact, that Coke and Doritos diet we discussed before—you may still encounter issues in the bedroom. As I often say, intermittent fasting will benefit you regardless of how you eat—but there are limits to what it can do.

Intermittent fasting has a powerful impact on testosterone level, raising it by 180 percent, and increasing luteinizing hormone, a testosterone precursor, by 67 percent. But longer fasting has the opposite effect, as a three-day or longer fast can lower it.[17] In addition, the reduced insulin level we discussed earlier, which is one of the key benefits of fasting, boosts testosterone level. This has dramatic effects on healthy erectile function. Another beautiful study conducted during the Muslim holy month of Ramadan showed that intermittent fasting raises the level of a hormone called adiponectin that makes you more insulin sensitive, which raises your testosterone level.[18]

There are some complicating factors that come with intermittent fasting, however. Ghrelin, the "hunger hormone" that stimulates appetite, also motivates us to find a partner and have sex. A higher level of ghrelin generally correlates with a higher sex drive; a lower level corresponds to diminished libido—in lab mice, at least. Adjusting your fast to reduce ghrelin-induced feelings of hunger could therefore tamp down some of your sex drive. Although few men or women report a reduction in desire due to intermittent fasting, most will feel less interest during multiday fasts.

Moving beyond physiology, one of the greatest influences on libido and sex appeal is confidence. Holding on to too much body fat lowers your testosterone level and decreases your libido, and it unquestionably eats away at your self-confidence. My old 300-pound self can attest to that. A pattern of fasting, sleep, and proper circadian health will reduce body fat, raise testosterone and human growth hormone levels, and boost sex drive.

What we all want, in the end, is to feel good about ourselves. We want to be in control. We want to know that we're experiencing our full potential or at least working our way there. Fasting and sleep, together, can get us there.

YOUR SLEEP MISSION

Even if you pay attention to your diet, cut out alcohol, give yourself some space from electronic devices, and attend to all the other habits of good sleep hygiene, sometimes you will still have a restless night. That's completely normal. With sleep, as with fasting, meaningful change and improvement don't happen instantly. You also have a real life with friends, family, work, and many other potential sources of worry and distraction. Give yourself time to adjust. Setting your expectations too high can make matters worse by adding to your stress.

Just as we've been programmed to believe the feeling that if you don't eat, you're going to die of starvation, most people have at some deep unconscious level enough fear of being tired that it causes anxiety. Let's rethink that. It's true that food and sleep are both essential, but it's also true that you're probably a lot more resilient than you think.

One of the training exercises for Navy SEALs is sleep deprivation: you get ten minutes of sleep, the trainers wake you up, they make you get up and put on a backpack, and then you run. The goal is to make you realize that you can do just fine even if you're exhausted. The military calls it sleep conditioning: you train your body to perform well in a nonrested state, even when your circadian environment isn't perfect. Emergency room doctors go through their own version of sleep conditioning. My wife is an ER physician, so I know the process well. Starting with their medical residency, ER doctors endure sleep deprivation until they learn to snap out of sleep and turn on their brain instantly to save a life. It's not optimal for anyone's health to endure sleep deprivation over a long period of time (remember, you can die from lack of sleep before you die from lack of food), but the training enables them to develop the confidence to do their job on remarkably little sleep. That reduces their fear of being tired, but unfortunately it also leads to higher error rates in their care. You want your doctors to have healthy circadian rhythms!

That said, you are both the medical savior and the elite soldier in your mission for self-improvement, and you should approach the job with the same kind of self-confidence. Be prepared to experience sleep disruptions, and know that they don't have to harm you any more than hunger does, at least in the short term. You should expect sleep disruptions in the early days of a prolonged fast. The first time it happens, it might be disorienting. You're going to wake up tired and feel unsure if you can make it through the day. Your irrational brain won't believe you when you say that your body will feel supercharged by the release of ketones and enough cortisol and adrenaline very soon—so that you may actually feel as though you've been reborn as a higher version of yourself.

Like hunger, sleep interruptions during prolonged fasting can create a stupid worrying voice in your head. Ignore it, or rather master it. It's okay if you get only four hours of sleep from time to time. I started Bulletproof while working full-time as a vice president at a big company on four hours or less of sleep per night, while also doing intermittent fasting and developing the Bulletproof Diet. I used fasting to help with my sleep deficits, and I used sleep hygiene hacks to keep my circadian rhythm on track as much as I could. All of these tools are available to you, too.

Get a full night's sleep if you can, and if you can't, relax and cut yourself a break. You're working to take better control of yourself, and you will never gain control by screaming and shouting. So when that stupid voice in your head yaps at you—"This is too hard, this is taking too long, I'm too tired, I'm too hungry, this isn't working"—don't yap back. Just remember your mission. You've got this.

6

FAST FOR FITNESS AND STRENGTH

On day three of the vision quest, I awoke still haunted by dreams of snakes. I instinctively searched my body for bites and examined the dusty floor around me, now illuminated by the sharp rays of the morning sun. There were no signs of slithering serpent marks. I was alive and starting to adapt to the sensations of solitude and now strangely reduced hunger. Well, for moments, at least.

From somewhere in my subconscious, I remembered a quote by the Stoic philosopher Marcus Aurelius: "If you are distressed by anything external, the pain is not due to the thing itself, but to your estimate of it; and this you have the power to revoke at any moment." Marcus Aurelius is better remembered as a Roman emperor who ruled from 161 to 180 CE. In Hollywood's stylizing imagination, he was the villain in the movie *Gladiator*. During his time in power, though, he also wrote a series of insightful Stoic essays. They were collected as the masterwork *Meditations*, which is where I came across that quote.

According to Stoic philosophy, emotions such as fear and envy are false, superficial impressions of the world. A sage (or a shaman?) who has attained moral and intellectual enlightenment should be able to see past them, rendering them impotent. Then that person can di-rectly pursue a life of virtue, the highest form of good and happiness. I wasn't thinking of myself as particularly virtuous at that moment, but I was feeling the first glimmerings of what it would mean to truly conquer my self-consuming emotions. Unfortunately, I was also still acutely feeling the physical limitations of my body.

By that point, I had shifted into an altered state—in large part be-cause, for the first time in my life, I'd been going without food for an extended period of time. And after all, I was sleeping in a cave used for spiritual ceremonies for centuries if not millennia. If you've never before fasted for more than a day, your body will try to inject thoughts of food into your brain ten times a minute, so that if there's any food nearby you'll take *just one little bite*. If your willpower wins out (or if there simply is no food around to tempt you), the body gets really angry. There's that voice again, booming in your head: "How dare you ignore me! Don't you know who I am? Think about cake! You're going to die if I don't get food. Hey, do you smell brownies?" I remembered that I'd eaten rattlesnake when I was growing up in Albuquerque and that I'd just missed getting to try fried scorpions one time when I was traveling in Beijing. Those would be my only local dining options. I was glad, though, that I hadn't sneaked that protein bar into my bag. My inner voice would have won.

As a former fat person, I knew that voice well. It's the same one that sabotaged me every time I'd lose twenty or thirty pounds, only to gain it back and then some. It's the one that wore out my willpower when I ultimately failed every diet I'd ever tried. Because I knew its power over me, though, I knew that if I was alone in a cave with no food, it couldn't win, no matter how pissed it got. I tried answering it with a voice of reason, drawing on the words of Marcus Aurelius. The hunger was driven by fear, I told myself, not by a genuine need. The reality is, you can go for a very long time without food. In general, it's going to take three months of eating nothing before you die.

The voice was lying, and I knew it. So no matter what your body tries to yell at you, it is just not true. I could safely ignore it and con-tinue to pursue my better self. I doubled my vow that I would finally achieve power over the voice of hunger. But my vision quest was far from over. The voices in your head that lie to you do not give up so easily. Did I mention that they were trying to convince me I was smelling brownies?

MASTER OF YOUR ELECTRONS

I want you to read this chapter with a stout heart, intellectual rigor, and a mind for truthfulness. Embrace the philosophy of Marcus Aurelius[1] (the Stoic part, that is, not the part with all the battles and throwing Christians to the lions, which had been fasted beforehand to make them extra ravenous). I want you to be able to look at what's on your plate—or what's not on your plate—and be okay with it. I want you to know that you are stronger than your fears and your cravings. I want you to know that your mind and body are full of untapped capabilities.

I want you to know that you're capable of exercising on an empty stomach and emerging smarter, faster, and stronger.

From our primal days 300,000 years ago, when *Homo sapiens* was the newest hominid species in Africa, all the way up to the present, we humans have cherished strength. It's how we survived in the wild. Sheer physical strength is no longer a daily matter of life and death for most of us, but being fit and active is still a measure of your ability to succeed and to enjoy the things you do. The importance of becoming stronger is built within us, starting at the subcellular level. The ultimate measure of strength is how many electrons your body can muster up quickly. So one of the first things your body does when you fast is get rid of the weak cells and grow more mitochondria—the metabolic power plants in the cells—through a process called *mitochondrial biogenesis*.

This regimen of cellular fitness training is the most foundational type of strength you can possibly have. When you fast, your ability to generate chemical energy increases. That improved efficiency allows your body to process even more fuel and generate even more energy. It's like pressing the accelerator in your car. How quickly can you get power to the tires? Well, the first thing you want to do is have an engine that's strong enough. Then you want to make sure that all the subcomponents delivering power from the engine to the transmission to the tires are also strong.

Fasting is like that. Intermittent fasting, in particular, strengthens your ability to deliver power, starting with the mitochondria and continuing up to the muscle cells, the neurons, the organs, and the body as a whole. When you get stronger at a subcellular level, you rebuild and improve yourself from the inside out. The end result is that you become stronger and more capable as a human being.

The other way fasting strengthens you is that it trains you not to waste energy. Ultimately, everything you think and everything you do is made possible by moving electrons from molecule to molecule. Fear and other negative emotions use up electrons. They direct your energy toward unproductive feelings and actions. Willpower uses electrons, too, so you want to apply it as efficiently as possible. Think of willpower as a mental muscle: you can exercise it. You can make it stronger so that you learn to fast and make it much easier to say no to cravings for muffins or potato chips or whatever junk you're better off without. Once you train the urges of the body to be more obedient, they ask for less energy. You waste less energy on fear and insecurity, and then you need to invest less energy in willpower. Those changes all make you more powerful in general. It is impossibly liberating to be able to smile at your hunger, then head to the gym and get twice the results from your workout because you made your body take the harder path.

This process of cellular and mental exercise improves everything from your spirituality to your resilience to your emotional state—all the way up to your physical toughness. The goal here is that you want to know you can handle whatever life brings your way. Only you know exactly what that means, but regardless of what you face or what you want to achieve, fasting will help you get there. It lets you demonstrate to yourself that you can take control, and it demonstrates to yourself that you must. You will get stronger through fasting. You will get stronger through exercise. And if you approach both of them the right way, you will truly optimize your strength.

But first, you may need to make some radical adjustments to your beliefs about exercise and food.

STRIKING THE RIGHT SUGAR BALANCE

My relationship with working out is long and still evolving. When I started gaining weight in middle school, I honestly believed that exercise alone would keep me healthy and make me thin. That's a flawed premise that many of us buy into. I played competitive soccer as a kid for thirteen years. Then I was a long-distance cyclist in mountain biking and road racing, entering a few races and completing several hundred-mile rides. I was only thirteen or fourteen and was doing the work, going the distance. And still getting fat and feeling like a failure.

In some ways, all that effort paid off. I enjoyed the training and discipline, constantly pushing myself to go farther and faster. But I was still gaining weight. There were things happening in my body that I just didn't understand.

Anytime you engage in endurance exercise—a routine such as a run or a bike ride that lasts an hour or more or even playing a long game of soccer that involves constantly running up and down the field—your body will eventually run out of fuel. Back then, I did what everyone else did, filling my water bottle with sugary "sports drinks" in order to power up and keep going. I would eat a banana with a little bit of salt or some electrolytes and lots of sugary stuff in order to fuel myself.

I had also read enough to know you were supposed to eat a lot of carbohydrates the night before a big physical event. Back in the 1980s, we called that strategy "carb loading"; you would eat an exorbitant amount of bread and pasta to fill your muscles with glycogen to use as fuel. If you didn't do that, everyone said, you would be susceptible to what we called "bonking." There's nothing sexual about that term; if anything, it's the exact opposite. Every endurance athlete knows what I'm talking about. Bonking is the terrible feeling that can happen when your muscles run out of the stored sugar in your body.

Believe me, you don't want to bonk. You start getting shaky. You have a feeling of nausea. You can't think. Your brain shuts down, and you just want to curl up into a fetal position. You feel as though you have no power output left. And it's not just an illusion. If you've never fasted, or if you haven't built up your metabolic flexibility in general, the bonk is reality. You're stuck, and the only thing that will unstick you is sugar. Your body doesn't recognize any other fuel source, and it will take about four days for your body to start producing ketones by itself if you start fasting right then.

Even if you tried filling up on a steak instead of sports drinks (assuming you could somehow find a steak in the middle of a hundred-mile bike ride), that wouldn't help with the bonking. If your body was trained to draw its energy from sugar, it will find a way to get that sugar. Eat a steak, and your metabolism will gladly transform protein into sugar on your behalf. Even worse, the dirty process of converting protein into sugar will unleash inflammatory by-products and lots of ammonia into your system. You'll feel better slowly—that is, until the next time your muscles run out of glycogen. In the long term, you'll also feel a relentless drag from all those toxins and inflammation.

Today, we have better approaches to staying well fueled during exercise. We have products such as stingers, gel packs, and energy chews. Stingers are small, crisp, honey-filled waffle sandwiches a cyclist or runner can ingest to keep his or her muscles topped off with glycogen. Honey is a sugary energy source that provides an instant energy boost. Gels and energy chews typically contain maltodextrin, a polysaccharide molecule that has an even higher glycemic (glucose-boosting) index than sugar. These things have their own shortcomings. Maltodextrin is derived from corn, rice, potato starch, or sometimes wheat, which can be a source of cellular inflammation. All three products rely on boosting your energy stores by using sugar or sugarlike products. There are also tons of sugar in all of the latest energy drinks. Whenever you eat sugar or carbs, your body will rapidly build up your glycogen store. It's a quick fix.

If you take in too much sugar, you will run into other troubles. You can store glycogen in two places: the liver, where it is rapidly available and will be used preferentially by the brain, and the muscles. For every gram of glycogen your body stores, you also retain roughly three grams of water. That's why heavy consumption of sugar and carbs produces a general look of bloating or puffiness. Beer drinkers know what I'm talking about. Your body has its energy and you feel good, but you haven't built up your fundamental strength. All you've done is tapped into a short-term boost.

You are better than that. Or at least you will be soon.

BODYBUILDING FROM THE MOLECULES UP

Fasting enables you to build up your metabolic strength, and one of the most basic ways to do that is to break your craving for sugar. Some people liken sugar to cocaine, because there is an addictive nature to sugar and both give you a dopamine hit. Both are proven temporary energy boosters, and they're both white powdery substances. The comparison is an oversimplification, but there is a kernel of truth in it.

Let's be clear, no one's doing lines of sugar. There isn't a sugar-smuggling mafia selling it for $1,000 a pound, or whatever the going rate might be for a kilo of cocaine. (It's not the kind of thing I keep track of.) On the other hand, look at the way the National Institute on Drug Abuse describes the effects of doing cocaine: "Small amounts of cocaine usually make the user feel euphoric, energetic, talkative, [and] mentally alert . . . and temporarily decrease the need for food and sleep." Side effects include a racing heartbeat, irritability, seizures, strokes, and coma. Sugar does all of those things, too, just in more subtle ways.

And just as coke addicts cannot live without their lines, sugar addicts are dependent on sugar. A lot of people are hooked on sugar, and we can see the social consequences clearly in our exercise patterns. Every time you get a little bit tired during a workout, you probably take a hit of sugar. Even if you don't exercise, you probably still keep taking regular hits of sugar. Managing fuel for short-term availability and short-term thinking has become our predominant metabolic strategy. There's some merit to the idea of carb loading the night before an endurance task such as a long bike ride, but life isn't a bike race, and the top racers today are starting their races running on ketones, not sugar! If you're eating like a 1980s endurance athlete every day for the rest of your life, all that sugar will wreak havoc on your body. It will make you weak.

Let's look at how you can become strong instead. What if you were to train yourself to switch effortlessly from burning sugar to burning fat? To most of the people at the gym, this probably sounds like a nutty concept. Sugar is energy. Fat isn't energy. How can you possibly maintain a high-impact workout powered by fat? Well, it turns out that you can definitely exercise at a high level, and in a major way, running on fat. And when you switch to burning fat, some very interesting things happen.

Fat molecules actually contain more energy than carbohydrate molecules. The good types of fat are also anti-inflammatory, which is especially important during exercise. By its very nature, exercise is pro-inflammatory. Physical exertion tears away at your muscle cells and activates an inflammation response. That is why you feel sore after a hard workout. If you look at the blood markers of someone who has just completed a marathon or who has just done a heavy lifting session to exhaustion, there are clear signs of inflammation.

That's not a problem, exactly. Inflammation is a natural and productive aspect of exercise. Your body gets stronger during the recovery cycle as it heals the inflammation and repairs your muscles at the cellular level. Muscle bulk is a by-product of that repair process. On the flip side, taking medication to reduce inflammation or even indulging in a simple ice bath halts this healing process and prevents muscular development. Even if your body aches the day after you do a hard workout, you're better off not taking ibuprofen: it's anti-inflammatory, so it's actually working against some of your goals for exercising. Let your built-in repair mechanisms work the way they evolved to work, and your body will not only fix itself but make itself stronger.

If you *really* want to assist those mechanisms, take sugar out of the equation and use anti-inflammatory fat as a fuel source instead. Then you will jump-start the healing and strengthening process. You'll be getting more energy and less inflammation at the same time. I was, to the best of my knowledge, one of the first people to stand up and say that it is possible to complete an Ironman triathlon in a state of ketosis, when the body is running mostly on fat-derived ketones. But there's a huge caveat: I also said that it is stupid to do an Ironman triathlon in ketosis. It's possible, but metabolically it's going to be damaging. I have the proof. I'm not allowed to name names, but I talked with the doctor of someone who did an entire Ironman—2.4 miles of swimming, 112 miles of cycling, and a full 26.2-mile marathon—while in ketosis. As I predicted, his lab tests showed that he was a complete disaster. Inflammation everywhere. Metabolism in shambles. Ketones and carbs at the same time? Rocket fuel! That's what I recommend.

The purpose of this book is to help you make the right choices with fasting, not take it to damaging extremes. Just because you *can* do something doesn't mean you *should*. That applies to life in general, and it applies to fasting in particular. The goal is not to suffer or to push yourself to the absolute limit. The goal is to make you better, more energetic, more confident, stronger all around.

A central element of metabolic strength is *metabolic flexibility*, the ability of your cells to switch quickly and easily from burning sugar to burning fat. The mitochondria in those cells already contain all of the chemical tools to make adenosine triphosphate, or ATP, your primary energy storage molecule, from either sugar or from fat, but most of the time only one set of tools is activated. The vast majority of us are locked into burning sugar, including the loads of sugar we get from breaking down carbohydrates. If your cells are stuck in sugar-burning mode, it makes it harder to lose weight and limits the amount of energy you have available.

Exercise and fasting create unpredictability for your cells. They get biochemical signals that sugar is available only some of the time; other times, they need to be ready to run on fat. They need to be prepared for anything. In response, the cells adjust their compositions and their structures so that either type of metabolism is ready to go. In addition to helping you with weight loss and energy gain, flexible cells do not develop insulin resistance and adapt easily to ketosis without making you feel lousy. By analogy, think about a phone that you can charge from a wall outlet but also from a cable in your car.

If you could charge your phone only one way, you'd be really limited. A phone that can power up wherever you go is much more useful, reliable, and enjoyable—just as you want to be.

FASTING AND EXERCISING TOGETHER

Now let's think through a smarter way to exercise using your own fat as your fuel, because ketones are anti-inflammatory and more energy dense than sugars and carbs.

Even as I write this book, I'm reading about Ironman triathletes, hundred-mile ultramarathoners, and other extreme endurance athletes who are learning to burn fat as they compete. They're not doing it in an all-out state of ketosis. Rather, they break their ketosis before or during the race with a small amount of carbohydrates. A minidose of carbs keeps their muscles filled with glycogen, but it also allows them to metabolize fat as a more potent fuel and hydration source. They train while in ketosis whenever they can, but they regularly exit ketosis and eat carbs and protein in order to raise their testosterone level. And then, when they are going to compete in an event, they start out the race with lots of glycogen and a metabolism that is happy to take energy from sugar or MCT oil and ketones.

Now, that is a regimen that I can endorse. It's an intelligent way to combine fasting and exercise to maximize their mutual benefits, the same way you learned how to combine sleep and exercise in the previous chapter. Start with a mild fast before you exercise, whether it's weights or high-intensity interval training. The best time to exercise is at the end of a fast, so for most of us doing intermittent fasting, it's around 1:00 or 2:00 p.m. After the exercise, when your body is primed to repair and build muscle, break the fast. Have some protein. Have some fat. If you want to exit ketosis, have some carbohydrate, too. Your workout will have been harder because you were fasted, but your results will be far greater, and the food will taste better after your workout.

If you're doing a long-endurance event, supplement your ketones in the form of C8 MCT oil—more than a few pro athletes use Bulletproof Coffee and amino acids such as L-glutamine. L-glutamine takes you out of ketosis, but it's quick energy, and your goal in a race isn't to stay in ketosis. Your goal is to have maximum energy from all pathways, including ketones, glucose, and amino acids. It's okay to have your favorite carbohydrate source, especially in the second half of the event. Your body is going to do better.

When your body burns fat, the carbon and hydrogen in the fat molecules combine with oxygen, which forms carbon dioxide and water. You breathe out the carbon dioxide, and your body makes use of the water, so you're actually hydrating your body as you go, the same way a camel stores water in its fatty humps. If you're competing in a long race and you've practiced fasting while training—but not necessarily during the race—your body will be better able to metabolize the energy you get from ketones.

Research backs up the effectiveness of this fat-first, fasting-enhanced exercise method. What you're doing is tapping into more of those chemical pathways that were shaped by millions of years of evolution. Enhancement of endurance through intermittent fasting was documented in a major study led by Krisztina Marosi when she was at the National Institute on Aging in Baltimore. "Evolutionary considerations suggest that the body has been optimized to perform at a high level in the food-deprived state when fatty acids and their ketone metabolites are a major fuel source for muscle cells," she and her colleagues concluded.[2]

Your challenge, then, is to become so resilient and flexible that you can start out with a full load of ketones and switch over to burning sugar. Intermittent fasting is the tool that will enable you to do that. The human body is built to burn sugar, or, if there's no sugar around, it will grumble for a little while, then start burning ketones from fat. In nature, ketones and glucose are never present at the same time. You can, however, trick your body into having both present at the same time using the wonders of supplementation!

Ketone supplements enable you to achieve ketosis without following a strict keto diet—that is, one completely devoid of carbohydrates. This works really well when you're metabolically flexible because your cells can use both fuel sources at the same time. One method is to put cold Bulletproof Coffee into your exercise water bottle but make it with very little if any butter. The MCT oil in Bulletproof Coffee raises ketones because it converts directly into the ketone known as beta hydroxybutyrate, or BHB, and it does so even in the presence of carbohydrates.

It's worth noting that there are companies that sell a product, ketone salts, that some athletes now put into their water bottles. They consist of BHB molecules that are bound to a mineral. I believe that taking ketone salts regularly is not a good idea. In the last interview he gave before he passed away, Richard "Bud" Veech, the world's most experienced ketone researcher, who studied ketosis for more than four decades, told me that ketone salts cause mitochondrial harm. Are they safe for short-term use, as during a race? Almost certainly. Do you want to take them regularly? Probably not. It's why I don't sell them. I'm similarly dubious about commercial supplements that contain ketone esters. In this case, the BHB molecule is bound to butanediol, an alcohol molecule that chemists use to make polyurethane. That doesn't mean ketone esters are bad for you—except that your body has to do some work to use them.

Ketone esters create a heavier load on the liver, and ketone salts take a load on the kidneys. I don't consider either one advisable for daily use. MCT oil is a perfectly natural source of ketones that is 100 percent biologically compatible. That's why it's a key part of the recipe for Bulletproof Coffee. If you need a bit of rocket fuel that doesn't have a metabolic cost and you use it carefully and occasionally, those alternatives could be acceptable. But I believe that MCT oil is a better and safer way to do it.

Ketone supplements work well for elite types of endurance events, but for overall strength and well-being what you really want to do is become highly resilient. You want to build up your innate strength so that you're equally powerful when you're on the basketball court or when you're in home isolation stressing about a pandemic.

Intermittent fasting sets you up for developing that kind of resilience. You go all night without eating. You wake up, drink whatever beverage you need for whatever type of fast you're doing: water, tea, black coffee, Bulletproof Coffee, whatever. Then, just before you're about to break your fast several hours later, you do your workout. You don't go for a long run. You could go to your strength trainer, work out with resistance bands at home, hop on your Peloton, whatever. You're not a masochist, after all. What you want to do is just a short fifteen- to twenty-minute, intense series of sprinting and resting exercises. This is known as high-intensity interval training, or HIIT.

The sprint-style workouts of HIIT have been around for decades, but it's only recently that science has shown the amazing fitness benefits they deliver. HIIT is the most simple, primal, and time-effective workout imaginable. A typical session goes like this: Sprint for fifteen to thirty seconds. Walk until fully recovered. Repeat. Do that for twenty minutes, if you can. Or up the game with seven to ten repeats of twenty seconds sprinting followed by just ten seconds of rest, which is a variation of HIIT known as Tabata.

When you run (or bike) at an all-out sprint, your body produces lactic acid, a by-product of burning glucose without enough oxygen present as it goes into oxygen debt. When your body produces lactic acid, it also produces copious amounts of adrenaline. This adrenaline directly corresponds with fat burning. In addition, a primal part of your being will panic as your muscles are depleted of glycogen. Your pancreas will release insulin into your bloodstream in an attempt to keep your body from starving. In time, this adjustment will enable you to metabolize fats and sugars far more efficiently. Although the workout is very brief compared with standard endurance workouts, the high intensity of HIIT (it's right there in the name!) means your body will continue to burn calories in the hours after the session is complete.

The research behind this is compelling. During HIIT, a component of fitness known as VO_2 (the volume of oxygen in the blood) is elevated and the release of certain enzymes is increased. VO_2 level increases during short-duration HIIT intervals are equal to those during a standard endurance workout of running and biking. In other words, you're getting a hormonal workout at the same time. A team of biologists at the Australian National University determined that HIIT boosts testosterone levels by 38 percent.

In their study, blood levels of human growth hormone shot up by 2,000 percent![3]

For you endurance junkies out there, it's worth noting that if you're training for a long competition, HIIT intervals are no substitute for a long run or bike ride, although for basic cardio fitness, there is research from the University of Colorado showing that two twenty-second high-intensity sprints on a bike produced exercise results superior to those of a forty-five-minute endurance exercise session on the same bike.[4] For endurance athletes, research has shown that elevating VO_2 is not as important as raising what is known as the anaerobic threshold, which is that personal red line where the body goes into oxygen debt. Either way, HIIT is an amazing way to increase your fitness without a major time commitment.

A short, intense workout unleashes the marvelous process of mitochondrial biogenesis. During biogenesis, the body increases production of ATP, the energy storage molecule in the mitochondria. This happens during endurance athletics, fasting—and, in this case, fasting with the addition of a HIIT interval. You know what it's like when the battery in your phone starts getting weak after you've had it for a few years? An analogous process happens to the energy storage pathways in your cells. Mitochondrial biogenesis rebuilds the molecular machinery that pulls the energy out of the ATP molecules. You are literally increasing the amount of available energy in your body.

HIIT is all about alternating fast and slow movement. Sprint as though a tiger is chasing you, then walk gently for a couple minutes at a pace much more slowly than you normally would, or for maximum results lie on your back and pant. Then sprint like hell again for twenty seconds: you can almost feel the tiger's breath on your back. Then walk very slowly for a couple minutes, and do it all again. Once you get used to the HIIT pattern, play around with your mental imagery to keep it interesting. Find your own make-believe pursuer. It never hurts to activate the amygdala's primal fight-or-flight response to make you sprint as though your life really depends on it.

If you do this routine near the end of a fast, even once a week, you'll be amazed at the results you get.

THE BATTLE OF CHANGE VERSUS CONSISTENCY

The body resists change because it takes energy. Left to its own devices, that means the voice in your head that says you'll starve if you don't eat cake will also tell you to just lie on the couch to save energy. The thing that scares your body the most is rapid change, because it could indicate a life-threatening situation. That intense reaction means you can use rapid change to grab your body's attention and cause your body to respond rapidly. In fact, the more rapid the change in inputs to your body, the more your body will respond. Therein lies a central paradox of human health: the body craves consistency (because it minimizes energy expenditure), but it also hates consistency (because it makes you weak). Exercise is a way to force your body to confront change, so that you can be strong.

HIIT works because your body has to go from 0 to 100 percent back to 0 percent in a short period of time. It's actually harder to do that than to go from 0 to 75 percent and stay there for a while. Fasting works because you go from eating normally to eating nothing and then eating normally again. It's more dramatic and harder than eating just 70 percent of the calories you need, but it drives far more positive biological change.

The same thing is true of weight lifting. Let's say my arm weighs ten pounds and I decide to go to the gym to add another five pounds of weight to it. That's not much of a change. I'm flopping around some puny five-pound dumbbells, trying to get bigger biceps, but nothing is happening. I burn a little energy, sure, but it isn't as though my muscle cells are really stressed by those measly five pounds of additional weight. It's time to switch to something far heavier. My new dumbbells weigh twenty-five pounds instead of five pounds, so I can exhaust the muscles in less time. As you'd expect, I see more gains in less time.

Thanks to this newly observed principle, which I call *slope-of-the-curve* biological response, you can consciously change the inputs to your system to be more dramatic, which saves you time and makes your body respond in ways it never would if you introduced changes gradually.

Another example of how you can create abrupt bodily change is a new method of strength training known as *blood flow restriction*, or BFR. You place inflatable cuffs, like blood pressure cuffs, around your upper arms and upper legs. Then you pump them up as you would a blood pressure cuff. They shouldn't be particularly uncomfortable, and they certainly should not cut off blood flow completely. (At that point, the BFR band becomes what is known as a tourniquet, and if you leave it on all day you'll end up losing a limb. You'll lose weight, but it's not the best way.)

After adjusting the BFR band properly with a hand pump, you exercise with almost no weight. You could even use those five-pound dumbbells. The crucial thing is that you've created a local hypoxic (oxygen-starved) state that switches your muscle cells into emergency mode. With BFR, you get the results of lifting heavy weights without having to put your ligaments and tendons under stress. You also cultivate a better cellular response. You're putting your cells into a state in which they're really panicking. The lack of blood flow and the resulting oxygen deficit activate all of their stress responses and their energy emergency mechanisms. Just as with HIIT training, the way to get the most out of BFR is to work out for a short period of time.

If you stack these things—fasting plus HIIT or fasting plus BFR—you ratchet up the intensity. The HIIT and BFR protocols work fine under normal dietary conditions, but they are even more effective during a fasted state. That trains your body to get its energy from fat and increases your metabolic flexibility. The more you exercise while fasting, the more you train your body to make a seamless transition between carbs/sugars and fat. If you do a HIIT or BFR workout at the end of your fast, though, keep in mind that it will not be your most vigorous workout. It will not be your fastest workout, either. But because it takes place while your body is already depleted of glucose, you will see great gains.

RUNNING HOT AND COLD

Here's one more way to get outsize effects from fasting plus slope-of-the-curve biology: hot-cold therapy. This one could hardly be simpler: you wake up in the morning and take a cold shower or do some other form of sudden cold therapy. Your body is startled by the temperature change and responds by unleashing all of the biochemical tricks it has to deal with a sudden challenge.

This is a condition known as *hormesis*, in which the body thrives by adapting to adversity. The idea is that you hit the body with a modest challenge or stress and the body actually overcompensates, getting stronger in the process. Medical researchers have found that cold therapy appears to have a number of impressive benefits, including pain relief, faster recovery from injury, better mood, a boosted immune system, and weight loss.[5] A regular ritual of cold-water immersion (whether through ice baths, cold showers, or plunges into a cold lake) has also been linked to a reduced risk of cancer and dementia, probably by strengthening the lymphatic system and circulation.

Note that you don't gradually cool the water to make it comfortable. You take your nice warm shower, and at the end, direct cold water at your forehead and chest, where your cold receptors are. Yes, it will suck—for exactly three days. After that, the sudden cold will drive the level of cardiolipin in your mitochondrial membrane up, enabling your body to generate heat more quickly. It will also burn more calories all day long.

After the cold therapy, if you feel ready for another shock, try hopping into a sauna, or at least switching the shower to hot again. The switch to heat is going to increase your blood pressure, increase your heart rate, make you sweat, make you detox, and raise your level of heat shock proteins, your inflammation-mediating molecules. Heat shock proteins are produced in response to stress and, despite the name, can also be secreted by the body when it is exposed to cold temperatures and many other forms of sensory assault. They're also not just a single type of protein but rather a whole family of protein molecules that protect against muscle wasting, making them a vital ally in antiaging.

The sauna will also raise your blood level of the molecule hypoxia-inducible factor 1-alpha, or HIF1A, which coordinates the biochemical response to an acute lack of oxygen. There are several other ways you can trigger HIF1A, including restricting blood flow, doing breathing exercises, or just holding your breath. By priming the HIF1A pathway in your body, that trip into the sauna has already prepared you for the oxygen-limited intensity of BFR training, a high-intensity interval sprint, or HIIT-style twenty-second sprints spread out over a five- or ten-minute period.

There is strong epidemiological evidence that sauna therapy is effective in halting cardiovascular disease and dementia.[6] Cardiologist Jari Laukkanen from the University of Jyväskylä in Finland (a country where saunas are practically a way of life) and his colleagues conducted a twenty-year study of middle-aged men who used a sauna regularly and found that the men who sat in the sauna for twenty minutes at least four times a week decreased their risk of sudden cardiac death and experienced a 40 percent reduction in all-cause mortality during the period of the study. The sauna fanatics also had a markedly lower risk of developing Alzheimer's disease.[7]

I should note that I first heard about infrared saunas in around 1998, before they were all the rage they are today. Back then, I was still seriously overweight and unhealthy; I had constant back pain and was inflamed all the time. In other words, I was desperate. I'd heard that a sauna could help with my symptoms, so I bought one of the early infrared sauna models available to consumers. You can learn from the long list of mistakes I made. I put the sauna in a corner of my living room, where it didn't really have a strong enough electrical circuit; as a result, I had a hard time getting it hot enough, and when it finally reached a useful temperature inside, it shut off. The safety measures that shut off a sauna after an hour are there for a reason: if you were to pass out in a sauna and it stayed on, you could easily die in what would become a slow cooker.

Fortunately, saunas have progressed a lot since then. The newer in-frared saunas heat up much faster and work much better. They toast you with a mix of far-infrared radiation, which penetrates and heats you on the inside, and near-infrared radiation, which warms mostly the surface of the skin. This combination may be especially effective for boosting your production of heat shock proteins. By the way, lap-top computers and cell phones are a lot more heat resistant than they used to be, so if you absolutely *must*, you can be on your phone in the sauna these days. (Full confession: I do regular Instagram Live events from inside my sauna. When my phone overheats, I run ice water over it until it comes back on. Thank goodness most phones are waterproof now.)

I'd prefer that you treat the sauna as a meditative place, but the really important thing is to find a system that works for you. If you have a busy life and the only way to make time for the sauna is by multitasking—then fine, go on your phone. I find that being in the sauna for thirty minutes isn't harming my day by taking away from my productivity, which it once did. Or maybe you want to take your devices into the sauna as part of your relaxation technique. Want to listen to audiobooks or podcasts? Do it! Do whatever makes your program of fasting, exercise, and body shocking fit your lifestyle.

My recommendation is that you master intermittent fasting first. Exercise on top of fasting. Try adding cold showers. Then experiment with an infrared sauna at a spa or at a friend's house if you are lucky enough to have a friend with a sauna. That will tell you if you really want to make the considerable investment of dollars, time, and space to have a sauna of your own. All I can tell you is that I bought one of the new, improved infrared saunas, and I have no regrets.

WHEN THE WORKOUT'S OVER

Fast. Exercise. Eat. That's the basic order of things as you are strengthening yourself. Which raises a big question: What should you eat *after* you exercise?

Your answer will depend on what you want your body to look like.

Do you want to look like an ultralean, strung-out endurance athlete? A "swole" body builder? Maybe not that extreme. It's better to find a comfortable middle: lean and muscular, not too much body fat, the picture of health. The look of health and longevity. I felt as though I had nailed it when the *New York Times* described me as "almost muscular." Goals!

It's all up to you, of course, but if I can make a suggestion, please avoid the starving animal look. This is the TV and movie version of what a fit person is supposed to look like. You know, the body aesthetic of Wolverine in the Marvel movies or of a woman who's single-handedly battling a battalion of enemy soldiers. That physique actually comes from actors fasting for two days and taking diuretics to get rid of the water from the glycogen that their bodies have been holding on to. The ripped, lean, sexy style isn't something you can actually sustain. It's just a temporary thing that actors and fitness models do to get ready for a shirts-off scene.

I promise you that they don't look like that all the time. It's a short-term fix and really unhealthy. In fact, I'll go further and say that it's unhealthy even to fetishize that body type. Just as Big Food tries to get you craving foods that you don't need and don't want, Hollywood fantasies get you craving a physique that would literally kill you if you tried to maintain it. This is another great opportunity for you to exercise more self-control. Try *going without* the helpless desire for the kind of body that no normal human has. Do some squats, and grow a nice backside. Do some leg lifts and get quads. Just don't expect to look like a superhero every day.

But I digress. Let's say that you want to put on some muscle or at least maintain the muscle you have. As soon as you're done lifting weights or doing HIIT intervals, you should eat. You can have some carbs as part of your postworkout meal. As I like to keep reminding you, it's okay even to have a little bit of sugar on occasion—just not a lot, because sugar is bad for you. If you decide to have some starch, choose something such as rice, sweet potato, or root vegetables. Take advantage of the fact that bumping up your blood sugar will release insulin, which will then help you put on muscle. Unending keto can make it harder to put on muscle. Cycle your fasting, cycle your keto.

Carbohydrates will also boost your blood level of a separate hormone called insulin-like growth factor, or IGF, which signals the body to put on muscle. You want to strike a delicate balance here, though, because a chronically high level of IGF is associated with colorectal, breast, and prostate cancer. This is a place where the yin-yang between diet and exercise really helps you. Over a long period, intermittent fasting tends to drive down your level of IGF, protecting you from its potentially disastrous health effects. But in the short term you can hack your metabolism to boost your IGF level temporarily, so that you can bulk up and build strength.

If you're not worried about being ketogenic and you want to put on muscle, you can also take an amino acid called L-glutamine. At the end of your fast—but only after you've exercised—take anywhere from 2 to 10 grams of L-glutamine. This flavorless powder will help you build muscle mass. It also supports a heathy gut lining and reportedly has a calming effect on your mood to boot.

Do you *have to* eat after an exercise session? Certainly not. If you're looking to push your metabolic limits as an extreme athlete or just to prove how strong you are, go ahead and return to fasting. It will push you into ketosis faster and help you lose weight, but you're going to feel pretty awful. But first you should make an honest assessment of your mental and physical state. Are you feeling strong? Confident? Directed? Or are you feeling overwhelmed? Remember that starting with an intermittent fast, exercising, and transitioning into a longer fast is very likely to raise your stress hormones. Having said that, if you're not already overstressed (from work and family and the news cycle and all the random things we all have to deal with in our lives), and if you're not sick, there's no obstacle. You can go ahead and undertake the fast-exercise-fast challenge.

It is perfectly acceptable to do a multiday fast and keep exercising during the fast, but not until you have adapted to fasting and exercising on shorter fasts. It's best to keep your workout basic. And don't exercise right before bed—which is never a good idea, honestly, because it raises your adrenaline levels and can interfere with sleep. During a long-term fast, you should go for a twenty-minute or longer walk every day. Your daily walking break will increase your lymphatic circulation, the cycling of resources through your immune system. It needs a little kick while you are you're giving your digestive system a break. Your body still needs to get rid of its toxins, even though you're producing less of them in the gut. The walk will refresh your immune cells and do wonders for your mitochondrial biogenesis. It's a simple, low-impact way to get stronger.

If you've reached the point where you feel truly powerful—rock solid in body and mind—you can go all-in on the attitude that you're going to do something hard every day. I'm talking about heavy lifting while you are also doing a long-term fast. Like running a marathon, this is a pretty dumb idea, but if you want to show yourself how strong you are, it's possible. There could be psychological benefits to feeling fully in control of your body. Just don't make a habit of it.

Let me warn you: You're going to really feel pretty darn tired. You're going to be dragging. You're going to be emotionally more reactive. You're going to be a little bit cranky. You're going to need a huge amount of sleep. Things that you would normally handle with no effort are going to feel bigger than they really are. The thing that sets you off might be a child whining, your boss telling you that you did a crappy job, someone cutting you off in traffic, or any one of a million other little things. Be prepared for them. Seemingly minor nuisances will loom large. You need to have the self-control to cut them back down to size.

If you are genuinely ready for the challenge, though, there are few feelings more exhilarating and life-affirming than pushing yourself harder than you've ever done before. Don't even think about it before you've built up your strength. But if your mind-set is that you're ready to show your body—and yourself—that you can do it, go right ahead.

You should do it because you want to do it, not because you feel you need to do it. This is certainly not something you want to do every time you fast, because it is incredibly depleting. If you must, try it once, and not more than once every few months. You can fast for multiple days every month if you want, and you can exercise lightly during those fasts.

However you choose to fast, however you exercise, and however you combine the two, keep your eye on the prize. What you're doing is finding the strength inside you in all the different ways you can interpret those words.

7

FAST FOR MENTAL AND SPIRITUAL HEALTH

The voice of hunger in my head couldn't make me eat in the cave, so it tried to find other ways to undermine me. After all, nobody knows your weaknesses better than you do.

I was now a couple days into the vision quest, sinking into the solitude of First Woman cave and retreating deeper and deeper into my own mind. Or maybe I was exploring outward. My senses seemed to be growing sharper, more vivid, almost unbearably intense. I became aware that the stone walls forming the canyon were not just red but dozens of distinct colors I hadn't noticed before. At one point I abruptly noticed that about a dozen sweat bees were with me in the cave. How had I possibly missed them before? I didn't know if they were the kind that stung or not, but almost everything in the desert will sting you. They definitely derived a perverse pleasure from circling my head. They distracted me so much that I almost didn't notice that I had way more energy than I'd expected.

At one point I left the cave and went for a long, slow hike, testing out that welcome strength while also seeking respite from the hunger and loneliness. I carried with me a talisman of sorts, a dark gray windproof fleece jacket that bore the names and heights of the mountains I'd visited that year: Mount Shasta in California, Mount Cotopaxi in the Andes, Annapurna base camp, and Mount Kailash in the Himalayas. It had a few holes from errant campfire sparks, but it was what I always wore when exploring. I still do. I also had my hair cropped short, keeping the style I had adopted during my spiritual travels in Tibet, and a manly beard suitable for a vision quest.

It was remarkable how far away I felt from the moment of arrival at Delilah's ranch. I laughed to myself, thinking back on it. She seemed unusual, for sure, but there was also something otherworldly about her. Every one of the few photos I had taken of her showed inexplicable orbs floating around her body. They looked like dust motes, but my lens was clean and they didn't appear around anyone else. When I wiped my lens and complained about them, she just laughed and said, "You really think those are dust?" To this day, I don't have a concrete explanation for what was showing up in those pictures, but Delilah demonstrated that she could cause more of them to appear on command before I snapped a new photo of her on my digital camera.

By the time I returned from the hike, though, my hunger had injected itself into my awareness again, and the water I drank to stay hydrated didn't seem to help. At least my stomach had stopped rumbling. But my mind began fixating on food again as those bees circled threateningly. I lay down to sleep for the night, feeling increasingly anxious. I had two more days to go without food, and I was truly on my own until then. My brain started fixating on survival strategies. Should I try to call on my Boy Scout training? Maybe I could harvest some wild prickly pear cactus and cut it open with a knife. Do people ever eat it raw?

Intellectually, I knew I was fine, but the voice kept telling me that my life was in danger. That being without food was an emergency. That's what hunger does to you when you don't know what to expect. I had not yet crossed over to a state of self-control. In fact, as the now-familiar darkness closed in around me once again, I was feeling very much out of control. The voice in my head began whispering about predators, but this time even louder.

Much louder.

The voice grew so loud and insistent that I swore I could hear the desert sounds of a predator coming for me. I became totally convinced that I might wake up with a mountain lion raking his three-inch claws across the soft flesh of my belly. Except that in order to wake up to an attack, I would have to be able to fall asleep first, and that night it didn't seem as though sleep would be coming to me.

WE ARE ALL SEEKERS

All of that fantasy and fear came from my brain.

We've talked about the ways that fasting can make your mitochondria stronger and your muscles stronger, reduce inflammation and extend longevity, help you sleep better, and even improve your sex life. We've talked, too, about enhancing the physical functioning of your brain, tuning its chemical balance and energy so you can think more clearly. These are all quantifiable, tangible changes. You can measure them scientifically. You can perform laboratory tests to confirm the release of specific hormones and ketones in the body that promote autophagy and improve your metabolic efficiency.

But you must also learn about the intangible aspects of fasting, because they are just as central to your well-being. In fact, they may be even more important, because they amount to the most basic reason for living. You could call it your *soul*. You could call it your *inner consciousness*. You could call it your *chakras*. Or your *midi-chlorian-powered Force*. Whatever terminology speaks to you, there is a deeply spiritual side to fasting. Many people would argue that all fasting has a spiritual dimension.

You might feel uncomfortable being asked to contemplate such a personal topic right smack in the middle of a book about intermittent fasting. Many people habitually keep their spiritual conversations separate from their conversations about the tangible world. For that matter, many people don't consider themselves spiritual or religious and don't necessarily see these things as important—or even serious.

I get where you're coming from, because that's where I started out. Bear with me.

I come from a long line of sober-minded folks. My grandmother was a nuclear engineer. My grandfather was a physical chemist who wrote for the *Encyclopaedia Britannica*. The two of them met while working on nuclear engineering projects at the dawn of the Nuclear Age. I grew up indoctrinated in the idea that humans are nothing more than meat robots—that I am a meat robot. Life is just a biochemical process of power in, power out. Too much power goes in, that means you ate too much. Not enough power goes out, that means you didn't exercise enough, therefore you get fat. Signals from your senses go into your brain, responses from your brain make your body move around and do things. Logic is all that matters. Anything that's not logical is therefore garbage and should be ignored.

Over time, I came to realize that this purely materialist view of human biology couldn't be true. Some of that revelation hit me while I was investigating various Native American traditions as a young man. A lot of it came later: in Tibet, in the cave in Arizona, in the jungles of the Andes, and in the process of getting married and starting a family. The whole point of spiritual practice, I see now, is that there's a lot of stuff going on inside us that is clearly just not logical. Consciousness is not logical, and emotions are not logical. (The voices that tortured me in the cave were definitely not logical.) We are not flesh and blood. Or rather, we are not *just* flesh and blood; we are much, much more than that.

Fasting is one way to discover this complexity. There's something inside you that is intimately tied to sensing and feeling rather than thinking. You intuitively know that hunger is a feeling, not a thought, and that feelings by definition are not rational. Some of the most powerful influences on your behavior aren't rational, so there is no way that you can manage them in rational ways. The art of fasting is teaching yourself when those feelings are real and should be acted on and when they're false cravings and impulses that are better put to rest. Fasting helps you gain the strength to act on only the feelings you choose to act on. It puts you into the driver's seat, which sounds great until you remember the first time you got behind the wheel of a car and didn't know where the brakes were.

Perhaps you still aren't on board with all of this. I'm not here to proselytize, I'm just here to help you gain productive experiences and skills. Use the scientific method. Observe, look at the evidence, and decide for yourself. Wherever you stand on more ethereal matters, I guarantee that you will experience altered states when you become consciously aware of your body's many unconscious behaviors around food. First you feel hunger, and then, before you really have a chance to think about it, there's something else. A twinge. A resistance. Something holding you back. An old program, well hidden. It's one thing to sit still and be alone or to meditate and become aware of your thoughts. What happens during fasting is that you become hyper-aware of all your senses. Sometimes meditation and prayer are about stilling the mind, sensitizing you to feelings, not thoughts. Fasting does that, too, but it also helps you dial into your instincts at a bodily level so that you can get a handle on the feelings that tend to divert you from the path you want to follow.

The simple act of denying your body food can be a significantly more expansive spiritual act than meditation or solitude alone. If you use fasting to deepen your faith or expand your consciousness—or even if you just keep yourself open to these possibilities—you will achieve much better results than if you focus narrowly on goals of weight loss or longevity. When you approach fasting this way, there is also a wonderful humility to it. If you're fasting for spiritual reasons, you probably won't make a Facebook announcement about your fast. The goal of spiritual clarity and renewing your faith is completely at odds with the dopamine hit of receiving "likes." You can make your fast a time of cleansing and transcendence that moves you beyond the triviality of modern culture. Better yet, you can just make spiritual fasting a part of *your* modern culture. The point is, if you ignore spirituality, you are missing out on an entire world of experiences.

Remember the importance of moderation in all of this. You can work your body too hard, and you can work your soul too hard. You don't want to get stuck in the group that says all fasting must be spiritual and you must put on a lily-white robe before you do it. There really are people like that. They missed out on the part about humility. Once you start running around in a robe, I'm not sure you're still keeping yourself open to new experiences, either. But you also don't want to get stuck in the group that refuses to keep an open mind and open eyes. As you are fasting, you may have a spiritual experience without intending to. Give yourself permission to make that journey, even if you don't think of yourself as religious or as a seeker. If you begin fasting with the thought "I am skipping meals purely for the physical benefits" and you end up having a profound spiritual insight, that's one hell of a bonus.

You can even regard your spiritual enlightenment as a purely scientific process, if you prefer. I've done meditation retreats in Nepal and Tibet and ayahuasca ceremonies in the Andes. Participants are always instructed to fast for a couple of days beforehand. Why? It's not just because you're going to throw up anyway from the exertion or altitude or fear—although that may be part of the reason. It's because it's what works, based on thousands of years of trial and error. Or it's because fasting puts you into a state of increased clarity due to ketones and what they do to energize the neurons in your brain. If you argue that spiritual experiences are just about chemistry and electrons, you can frame it this way: deep concentration requires more electrical output from the neurons in your brain, and the neurons prefer ketones to glucose because of their greater energy density. Ketones have more electrons than glucose. More energy, more brain activity, more consciousness.

In other words, the spiritual side of fasting happens in conjunction with the scientific side. They are not two separate things. Advanced spiritual states are mentally demanding, so they are also metabolically demanding. You can marshal extra energy through specific diets that remove the toxins that are slowing you down, or you can remove those toxins through fasting. (Ideally, you'll do both.) In addition, you can use fasting as a spark to release the latent chemical energy your ancestors would have used to survive: for the final sprint in a hunt or for the last surge to go find some sort of sustenance. When you need that energy to take you to a new level of consciousness, you're going to have a much easier time getting there if your body is strong and metabolically fit.

Fasting strengthens your connection to other people as well, because whether we have a billion dollars or nothing at all, we've all experienced the feeling of hunger. When we see someone who is hungry because he or she has no food, we reflexively feel his or her despair. In fact, there are cells in the brain called mirror neurons that attune us to other people's emotions just by our observing their faces. And the more we fast as a spiritual practice, the greater our access to a deep reserve of empathy and connection becomes. The more we are able to transcend the needs of the self and quiet the persistent voices of the ego, the more we are able to tap into our sense of belonging in the larger collective.

Our shared humanity is defined by more than the common material needs of survival. We all share a hunger for purpose—for a way to put our constructive imprint on the world—and fasting brings out this hunger every bit as much as it brings out the more literal, physical kind. When someone chooses to abstain from food for spiritual reasons or to explore what makes him or her tick, it inspires us to do the same. On a practical level, once you are stronger, you will have more capacity for doing good in the world. You will be more able to solve problems and provide skills and resources that will benefit the people around you. Fasting truly reinforces our imperative to connect in so many ways.

In my travels through Nepal and Tibet, as well as in my personal studies and my experience fasting with the shaman in Arizona, I've learned firsthand that fasting is inherently both a physical and a spiritual process. The ultimate source of your focus—whether it is on meditation, on God, or on your next burger—is the neurons in your brain. They want ketones. When you start fasting, those neurons stop burning low-octane glucose and start devouring the new high-octane fatty molecules. You gain clarity because there's more of a spark inside your brain. More energy. For most of us, it takes a lot of effort to achieve such a spiritual state; it generally doesn't happen when you're overfed and exhausted.

THE JOY OF *GOING WITHOUT*

The reasons people undertake a spiritual fast are varied and deeply intimate: renewing their faith, mourning the death of someone they loved, emerging from a life crisis, recovering from addiction, searching for purpose. No one can tell you the right reason to do it. Your motivation is something that belongs to you alone. What I can do is offer some guidelines, drawn from my own hard-earned experience, about how to mentally prepare for an effective spiritual fast.

First off, embrace the joy of fasting. When people hear the words *spiritual fast*, they often picture ascetics who have removed themselves from society and deprived their bodies of all enjoyment. In this imaginary scene, the ascetics are probably flagellating themselves madly in the hope that physical pain will help them atone for indiscretion or weakness. Think of that as the old-school spiritual fast. It's not how I roll. (If I want to inflict suffering on myself, I'll just eat some kale.)

Fasting is not about pain; it's about discipline, self-control, and self-improvement. You may choose to push your limits—and it's not my job to tell you what limits to push or how hard—but pain is a distraction from the transcendental awareness you're seeking.

Second, you can do whatever you want during a spiritual fast. You can have sex. You can dance. You choose; it's up to you as long as you maintain a focus on spiritual awareness. The point is to make your body go without food, not without pleasure. The Tantric and Daoist schools teach that ejaculation is depleting. If you're a man, it really is much better to have as much sex as you want during an extended fast but not to go all the way until you finish the fast. The same teachings say that if you're a woman, you should feel free to climax as completely as you possibly can. Science now shows that there is a real drop in testosterone the day after ejaculation, which will indeed make you irritable.

I didn't believe any of this. I read about it and set about conducting an experiment to disprove it. For an entire year, I graphed the frequency of ejaculation and sex plotted against my happiness levels. I published the graph in an earlier book showing that happiness reliably falls the day after ejaculation—call it an ejaculation hangover, just for men. The lesson here is more nuanced. If you're on a spiritual (or normal) fast, you're already pushing yourself. You may be crankier and have less energy. You simply don't want to deplete yourself further, because the next day your willpower to resist food or resist yelling at your boss, your spouse, or your kids, will be lower. Why suffer more when you're fasting?

If you're a man and you ignore this advice, expect an epic orgasm, because your brain will be powered by ketones and you will be in a slightly altered state. It's just that you'll regret it in the morning. If you're a woman and you have sex during an extended fast, your orgasms will likely be more intense as well. You don't read about it often, but both men and women can have intense spiritual visions during orgasm. Sex and fasting together make it far more likely.

That said, just snuggling in bed can make fasting easier because it will raise your blood level of oxytocin, a hormone associated with love and social bonding. Just don't finish. Sorry, that goes for masturbation, too. I know, this is a sacrifice, but your momentary loss of seismic pleasure will be offset by the ways that an effective fast heightens your sense of arousal and connection to those you love. Your improved mood and increased energy could lead to a more profound and powerful sex life over time, and a stronger relationship with your partner in general.

Third, avoid self-judgment during your fast. Think of it this way: your physical fast cleanses the body of chemical impurities, while your spiritual fast cleanses your consciousness of the emotional baggage that weighs you down. These are not easy jobs! We all have some spiritual toxins in need of cleansing, and the mental clarity that comes with fasting may shine a light on problems you didn't even know you had hidden away. You may become aware of aspects of your personality, or perhaps memories or motivations, that are holding you back. This awareness will pull you further along the spiritual path. It will help you see the person you want to be and then will draw you along toward realizing that vision. I find it useful to keep a journal to record these observations.

While you're learning to fast, it may well happen that you break the fast and then regret it. Sooner or later, everyone who fasts regularly will have a time when they resolve to fast for two days, say, but something in their mind convinces them that it's a fantastic idea to break the fast early. Very quickly, you come to understand that there's someone other than you inside your head calling the shots. It's a very persuasive voice, capable of convincing you that it's your idea to eat a cookie in the middle of your fast.

There's a name for that voice: it's your *ego*. Learning to face down your ego and transcend it is the goal of spiritual practice. Fasting is going to make your ego scream that you're starving, even though you know damn well that your body has plenty of energy available. Fasting helps you perceive what is actually happening, stand up, and take charge. As you go on your own journey, just like my walk with the shaman, keep in mind that no one is perfect. No one succeeds right away in every effort to change. Simply being on that journey, actively engaged, is enough.

Sometimes, you will eat the cookie. That's okay.

TRIPPING ON OXYGEN

Here's a fourth major guideline to assist you in your fast. Whether or not you are focusing on the spiritual aspect, adding breathing exercises will bring more oxygen to the fire. After all, whether you're in ketosis or burning sugar, your body makes energy by combining air and food to generate electrons. When you alter your style of breathing—*boom!*—you can modify the other side of the equation, adding oxygen to speed metabolism or holding it back to build cells strong enough to thrive with less food *and* less oxygen. You're already burning fat by virtue of fasting. If you have less food, you can deliver more air and still have an abundant supply of energy. Your body is always trying to keep the equation balanced. At the end of the day, you can accomplish your goals in a low-oxygen, food-rich environment, or you can do the same in a high-oxygen, low-food setting. It all depends upon how you play around with the variables.

If you bring more oxygen to bear on your spiritual practice, all of a sudden things will change. Controlled breathing, in addition to fasting, is a part of many religious and meditative practices. One example is pranayama breath work in Hindu practice. Defined literally, it comes from an ancient Sanskrit word that roughly translates as "breath exercises." My introduction to this practice came years ago, shortly after I met my wife, when she perceptively told me, "You should start doing yoga." I took her advice and discovered that most of the classes ended with pranayama breath work. Some of the techniques seemed disarmingly simple, such as doing guided breathing while covering one nostril and then the other, but they led me to some really surprising altered states. That was a big discovery for me, just how malleable consciousness is.

That was also when I came to appreciate the enormous variety and complexity of breathing techniques. Most of us believe that deep breaths are good for us, healthy and relaxing. There's just one problem: taking lots of deep breaths and breathing more reduces the amount of carbon dioxide, or CO_2, in your body. You can hold only as much oxygen in your body as CO_2. That's why hyperventilation makes you dizzy. In fact, blood flow in the brain decreases when you breathe deeply or quickly. The ancient breath practices therefore generally focus on slower breathing—basically, taking reduced breaths; slower breaths, not deeper.

Slow breathing into your diaphragm stimulates the vagus nerve, the longest nerve in the peripheral nervous system. The vagus nerve is a vital communication highway that connects the brain, heart, and liver. Messages carried along the vagus nerve serve to regulate everything from speech to digestion to body temperature. One of the most significant roles of the nerve is in controlling blood pressure. If your blood pressure is too high, the vagus nerve sends signals throughout the body to lower your heart rate, bringing forth a sense of calm while reducing stress, anxiety, and anger. Stimulating the vagus nerve via diaphragmatic breathing, or deep breathing, sweeps away these potential impediments to a successful fast. Even if you are not actively seeking a spiritual state, you will not enjoy your fast if you're feeling edgy and anxious.

You can create a sense of calm by breathing in slowly, then making a very long, slow exhalation, over and over. At the start of each breathing cycle (the inhale) your sympathetic nervous system slightly elevates your heart rate. During a prolonged exhale, your vagus nerve does a most marvelous thing, sending out a message that overrides that temporary instant of panic. By releasing the neurotransmitter acetylcholine, the vagus nerve slows your heart rate. A prolonged exhale enhances vagus nerve function, lowering stress levels and improving cognition. Psychologists Roderik Gerritsen and Guido Band at Leiden University in the Netherlands developed a biophysical model suggesting that the response of the vagus nerve is directly related to the euphoric and otherworldly effects of yoga and meditation.[1] That insight suggests another biohack for fasting: when you feel hungry, take a few slow, deep breaths into your diaphragm, which will tell your body to calm down.

Another form of breath work that can accompany a spiritual fast is holotropic breathing, a body control technique for attaining elevated consciousness that was developed by the Czech psychiatrist Stanislav Grof as a way to mimic the effects of LSD without taking drugs. Stan is widely credited as the father of transpersonal psychology, which applies the techniques of therapy to the pursuit of spiritual enlightenment. When I first tried it, I was shocked by how much I could alter my perception of reality merely by manipulating the flow of air into my lungs. Holotropic breathing uses very fast, deep breaths for a short period of time to launch you into an altered state for healing. You don't have to be fasted for it, but it is more effective if you are in a fasted state or if you provide some ketones through a dietary hack.

Doing holotropic breathing[2] with Grof, I've had some wild experiences. I've left my body. I've seen what looks like past lives. People who believe in past lives say that when you experience one, often the first thing you see is your feet in the past life. As I lay on a mat in an old hotel in Palo Alto (which has now been replaced by condos), I breathed until my hands and feet tingled. Suddenly, I was aware of feet that weren't mine but at the same time belonged to me. I looked around and entered an intense vision of a life about six hundred years ago. In that vision, the man with the strange feet died with just one regret: that he hadn't finished training one of his students. When the breathing was done, I sat stunned, as I realized I knew someone in my life who reminded me of that student. Feeling stupid, I tentatively told that person, "I had a weird vision of a past life, when you were my student. Sorry I had to go before I was done." The impact on my friend was immediate—like being punched in the gut, followed by an enormous outpouring of grief. My vision connected to a highly private memory from my friend's past, something he had never shared with me.

I don't have the tools to explain it, and there's no way to verify that it's anything other than a hypoxic state generating visions. It sure didn't *feel* that way, and it doesn't explain why two sentences summarizing it would create that response in another person. I'm still mystified to this day, but I choose to believe that it's more likely real than not.

In fact, I've seen more through holotropic breathing than I have through experiencing ayahuasca. You can have experiences like that, too. Some people practice it alone, but that's not for the faint of heart. I recommend that you find an expert in holotropic breathing and try it when you are doing a spiritual, contemplative fast. You won't be sorry. You can do it without drugs, without danger—while you are doing things that improve your health, in fact. This type of breathing is yet another reminder that you are a lot more than the bag of meat you walk around in.

There are many other breathing techniques you can experiment with as well, and nearly all of them work better with fasting. There is the Wim Hof method of breathing, developed by the Dutch extreme athlete of the same name, which will give you superpowers for handling cold showers or ice baths, with or without food in your system. Or there's the popular "Art of Living" technique, which focuses on full yogic breaths and abdominal breathing. I did it every morning for five years before falling out of the daily practice when I moved and had kids. An estimated 40 million people do Art of Living daily.

All of the heavy-duty breathing methods I've discussed so far can be used in conjunction with fasting to deliver even more profound results. Fasting makes your metabolism more powerful, and that power requires oxygen to reach its full potential. For spiritual fasting, especially when you're getting started, the breathing method I prefer is one developed by the world-renowned integrative physician Dr. Andrew Weil. It's simple and easy. His method is called the *4-7-8 technique*, and it's just as simple as it sounds: Breathe in through your nose for four seconds. Hold the breath for seven seconds. Then breathe out for the count of eight, expelling all air from your lungs and making an audible "whoosh" sound as you do so. You should repeat this cycle up to four times in sequence and do it twice a day. During a fast, you can increase the number of repetitions up to as many as twelve. Dr. Weil has found that the 4-7-8 technique is ideal for helping you fall asleep at bedtime. During fasting, it reduces cravings and anxiety and helps control mood swings.

Everybody should know basic controlled breathing methods. They have the effect of calming the body, centering the mind, and focusing energy. It may take some time and practice to master breath work and see the benefits—as I've said, it's not easy for most of us to access a spiritual state. Learn to fast first. Then learn to breathe. The spiritual feeling will follow.

It's common for people to regard spiritual energy and biological energy as two distinct things: one subjective and personal, the other objective and (in some mysterious sense) absolutely "real." That distinction is an artificial one, though, as misleading as the idea that we are just meat robots.

Your body has a tremendous amount of distributed operational intelligence, meaning that your brain doesn't need to tell every cell in the body what to do. Your cells go about their jobs independently and then report what they did or didn't do in the form of electrons. Biology textbooks will tell you that the signals are carried by molecules such as peptides and hormones, along with electrical currents and probably even magnetic currents. Whatever terminology you prefer, our internal communication system is fundamentally all about moving electrons. By the time the signals reach your conscious mind, they've been heavily processed and filtered by a bunch of cells that did their job and didn't bother telling us about their little accomplishments.

When you experience a lack of oxygen in the brain, like the state of hypoxia you enter with holotropic breathing, you become suddenly, often psychedelically, aware of all that lower-level activity. Your brain cells selectively and elegantly start trimming the least urgent jobs on their to-do list. All through the body, your mitochondria will note the lack of oxygen for making energy from food, and your cells will cut back on the nonurgent tasks of digestion and detoxification. You're still not aware of the specific changes going on, but you sure can feel the effects. You relax, because your body is cutting back on its internal work. A lot of the conserved energy is directed to the brain, to make sure you survive. You feel fewer distractions, and you are able to access altered states more easily. Basically, your brain doesn't have enough energy to maintain some of the illusions you believe in.

Now you have the basic tools and the basic understanding to do a spiritual fast. Control your food, control your sex, control your breathing, and do it all from a place of wonder and ecstasy, not from a place of fear and suffering. To that end, remember: these things take time. If you're a brand-new faster, you're going to have a hard time pushing through the hunger, just as I had a hard time in that cave. Your little monkey mind is going to be running around going, "I'm going to die. I'm going to die. What's for lunch? *What's for lunch?*"

Do a few intermittent fasts before you go on a spiritual fast. You will feel triumphant when you put your monkey mind in its place. Then when you're ready to do a longer, spiritual fast, you will have the training you need for a more profound experience. All the life energy that was going into digesting your food is now yours to direct to a higher purpose.

MAKE ME ONE WITH EVERYTHING

I don't practice a specific religion, but I've done a lot of spiritual exploring. I've meditated. I've participated in many different religious ceremonies. I've done basic shamanic training with Alberto Villoldo, the founder of the Four Winds Society in California. Now I have young kids, so I've incorporated spirituality into our family rituals: all of us have a daily meditation practice and a daily gratitude practice for food. There's zero doubt in my mind that if you fast for a day or two, you'll have more spiritual experiences than you would if you spent the same time eating peanut butter sandwiches. You may also gain a more vivid experience of the world, possibly more vivid than you've ever known. Remember the story of my friend Chris, the army guy who said he could smell a hamburger from two miles away when he was deprived of food? I know that's not an exaggeration, because I experienced something very close to that in the cave and on other fasts since then.

Go for a walk in the forest when you are immersed in a fast, and observe the woods around you. Everything is a different color than you remember it being. The leaves on the trees are vibrantly green. Your senses are wide open. Most of the time we sit with our senses partially closed off, because we don't need all of the information they have to offer. We already have more food than we need and more information—more distractions—than we need. When you do a spiritual fast and you spend some time in nature, the whole world's a different place.

It reminds me of a story about a group of explorers who traveled into the remote wilds of Tibet, to the valley where the legendary Shangri-La is supposed to be located. Only a few Westerners have ever been allowed to go there. The explorers made many trips before the local guides would agree to show them where to go. But there was one doubter in the group—an asshole, to be blunt. When they finally arrived at the sacred location, that one looked around and snorted, "This is just a mountaintop. I don't see anything here." The local Tibetan lama who had guided them just smiled and responded, "Yes, you wouldn't." Meanwhile, the other explorers had a transcendent experience. You can choose to make fasting a slog to suffer through or a gateway to something bigger.

Fasting changes your perception of the world. That's why it has a place in almost every spiritual practice and religion. In the Muslim tradition, fasting is one of the Five Pillars of Islam. The celebration of Ramadan each year is a spiritual milestone, with fasting as a cornerstone. During this month of spiritual reflection and devotion, the daily fast goes from dawn to sunset. Muslims perform a dry fast, meaning they do not even drink water, in the belief that it cleanses the soul from impurities and encourages greater self-discipline and sacrifice. Each morning before dawn during Ramadan, they consume a small meal. More than a few Muslims have told me that Bulletproof Coffee is a big part of that meal. Then each evening, the fast is traditionally broken by eating dates, followed by a larger meal.

In Zen Buddhism, fasting is historically a requirement to reach some of the altered states that occur during advanced meditation, such as Samadhi. Because my 40 Years of Zen company offers advanced meditation with neurofeedback, I have had the opportunity to combine neurofeedback with fasting and reached a state where I became one with everything, for lack of better words. It sounds goofy, right? Like the old joke where the Zen master walks up to the hot dog vendor and says, "Make me one with everything." But I lived that experience.

During a particularly arduous two-hour session of pushing my brain to align its brain waves, I was getting exhausted. Suddenly my arms disappeared. I don't mean they went numb, they were just . . . gone. Not in a scary way, not painful, just curious. Then the feeling spread from my arms to my torso and my legs, and suddenly I realized I had no body at all. What I had thought was my body had dissolved. To this day, I remember what it felt like when my physical self was smeared across all of space. Now, about 80 percent of people who use the technology have a transcendent experience, according to internal research at 40 Years of Zen, but we give them C8 MCT oil instead of having them fast so they can do more.

Would my early beta-testing experience have been even more profound if I had some MCTs in my body at the time? Probably, to be honest. There is always a higher state to seek. But I don't think I'd have had the experience if my gut had been full of pizza.

Hinduism features a practice known as *vratas*, which involves complete and partial fasting. Different deities have different fasting days. For instance, Shiva requires a Monday fast, while Vishnu's fast is celebrated on Thursdays. According to the Jewish and Christian traditions, meanwhile, Moses fasted for forty days, according to the Book of Deuteronomy in the Bible. In the Book of Samuel, King David fasted to beg God to save the life of a child. Fasts were proclaimed during times of calamity and injustice, as noted in the Old Testament books of Jeremiah and Joel. Very often this was done throughout a particular kingdom as a means of drawing attention to an outrage, so that the voice of the people might be heard. In Psalm 35, King David declared that "I humble myself through fasting."

Biblical fasts were of two natures. One was known as an "absolute" fast, three days of no food or water. The other was the "supernatural absolute" fast, which was forty days without food or water. (No modern human has been recorded going without any food or drink at all for forty days, which is what makes it definitively supernatural.) Moses undertook two such fasts, one of which resulted in his leaving the Israelites to be closer to God at the top of Mount Sinai. He returned with the Ten Commandments, which were inscribed on two stone tablets. "Moses was there with the Lord forty days and forty nights without eating bread or drinking water. And he wrote on the tablets the words of the covenant," reads the Book of Exodus.

The Bible also speaks of a partial style of fasting, the Daniel fast. This involved abstaining from certain foods for a certain length of time. The New Testament's Book of Daniel tells of how he once fasted three weeks on vegetables alone, eschewing juices, meats, wine, and even body lotion. At the end of the fast, which coincided with a period of mourning, he witnessed a vision of a man with a "face like lightning, his eyes like flaming torches, his arms and legs like the gleam of burnished bronze, and his voice like the sound of the multitude." Daniel was with a group of men at the time, standing on the banks of the Tigris River in what is now Iraq. No one else could see his vision. When the flaming man spoke, he told Daniel that his fast had allowed him to "gain understanding and to humble yourself before God." No matter how you interpret the vision by the Tigris, it's clear that fasting and revelation have gone hand in hand for thousands of years.

Today, Jews still fast annually on Yom Kippur, a day of spiritual and physical cleansing when people ask forgiveness, grant forgiveness, and make plans for self-improvement in the coming year. Fasting is part of the Roman Catholic and Eastern Orthodox traditions during the annual celebration of Lent. In modern practice, people observing

Lent abstain from meat on Fridays and reduce the size of their other meals. The Lenten fast used to be a lot more intense, however. The "black fast," which continued the entire forty days and nights of Lent, once consisted of just one meal a day, eaten only after sunset. Meat, dairy products, eggs, and alcohol were completely forbidden. During the last week of Lent, the fast was even more strict, with salt, bread, herbs, and water the only foods allowed.

Hildegard von Bingen, the renowned twelfth-century Benedictine abbess, composer, philosopher, and mystic, created a beautiful spiritual elaboration of the Church's medieval fasts. Her fasts often lasted six to twelve days, beginning with a period of controlled breathing and meditation, and were intended to foster a sense of unity and balance. Her spiritual fasts were built around rest, meditation, a regular daily time to explore spirituality through prayer and journaling, intervals of solitude, and time spent in nature. She was an acute observer of nature, writing influential books on the properties of plants, animals, and the local geology. She was quite far ahead of her time!

One quibble: Hildegard allowed bone broth during some of her fasts. I would avoid that because the broth contains protein that will disrupt your fast. But this was more than eight hundred years ago, so let's cut her a break.

The stern version of Lent began to change in the fourteenth century as the Catholic Church loosened its rules on fasting, and religious fasting practices continue to evolve to this day. The importance of fasting for proper observance remains a constant, however. Many modern Catholics still maintain a black fast on Good Friday and Ash Wednesday, which is basically OMAD combined with a protein fast. If anything, the practice of fasting for spiritual growth is gaining popularity among mainstream religious groups. The Saddleback megachurch in southern California, one of the United States' largest Christian congregations, has created the Daniel Plan, a set of dietary guidelines based on the food choices made by the biblical figure Daniel. Spiritual fasting is a key component of the plan. I have a special fondness for this approach: Dr. Mark Hyman, a specialist in chronic illness and longtime friend, played a key role in the development of the Daniel Plan.

THE GREATEST FAST OF ALL

Spiritual fasting can take you to some terrifically unusual and un-expected places. I mean, Daniel in the Bible saw a guy with flam-ing eyes. Hildegard of Bingen had a vision of a woman with a scaly monster sticking out of her belly.[3] I had a hallucination of murderous mountain lions. But I have had other ethereal and inspiring expe-riences when fasting that connected me to realms for which there are no words. I left them with more resilience, more certainty, and a greater sense of my purpose. Who knows where you will go with your fasts? Just know that fasts, especially longer than forty-eight hours, may take you to some new places if you let them. You are also per-fectly capable of going to work and living normally while fasting for the same period of time.

The more you can move your life obstacles out of the way, the richer your spiritual experience will be. Sometimes a spiritual fast does not involve abstaining from food but instead a separation from the distractions of the material world. Normally when you're fasting for meditative purposes, you intentionally schedule your fast for a time when you won't be superbusy. You slow down and deliberately go without distractions. You're really adding another layer of *going with-out*: you're doing a moderate version of a dopamine fast, the stimulus reduction plan described by my friend Cameron Sepah at the Univer-sity of California San Francisco.

For thousands of years, traditional religions have understood the value of abstaining from things other than food. During Yom Kippur, for instance, Jews are forbidden to wear leather or perfume, bathe, and have sex. Lent and Ramadan likewise are times when observant people turn away from material goods and easy pleasures. The Sab-bath embodies many of the same ideas on a weekly basis; it is the reason that liquor stores are not open on Sundays in some places.

This type of fast is sometimes known as "fasting from indulgence," and it is an attempt to deepen a spiritual connection, with or with-out an accompanying fast from food. It might include spending less time shopping and doing work or spending time in nature instead of staring at your phone. Such acts of *going without* are the essence of a spiritual fast: they unburden you from worldly distractions and open the possibility of greater understanding, a greater connection with a higher power, and a fresh perspective on where we stand in relation to the universe.

We've now looked at quite a number of different forms of *going without*. But really the most challenging type of fast that you'll ever do is the one that I'm still working on today. I've managed to stick to this fast sometimes, but not all the time. It's *fasting from hate*.

Try spending a day without thinking hateful thoughts about anyone or anything. It's far, far harder than spending a day without unconsciously eating something in the middle of a fast. Remember the four F-words that drive all life? The first one is *fear*. Hate is what we do when we can't run away from, hide from, or kill something that our primitive animal mind believes is a threat. Hate is the source of so many current troubles in the world. It is what divides us into tribes at voting booths and on social media. It is the mind killer that makes you think in absolutes. It is at the root of gaping inequalities in economic opportunity, health care, education, and justice. Hate tears apart families and friendships. When you decide to fast from hate for a day, you will see the disturbing truth that it is everywhere. Social media memorializes our hate when we have a momentary emotional outburst and makes it easy to hate other people online. Whether you decide to put down your fork for a day or to forgo hate for a day, you have stepped onto the path of liberation, self-improvement, and self-realization.

The point is, all of the different forms of fasting support one another. If you can succeed in fasting from hate, you'll find you have more compassion for yourself even if you do end up eating the cookie that you promised yourself you wouldn't eat. You'll begin a journey toward forgiveness—and you'll notice that forgiveness is one of the core elements of every major religion and spiritual system.

That's the challenge and the great potential here. Fasting in all of its forms teaches you to be less judgmental of yourself. From there, you can learn to be less judgmental of others. Change yourself, change the people around you, change the world.

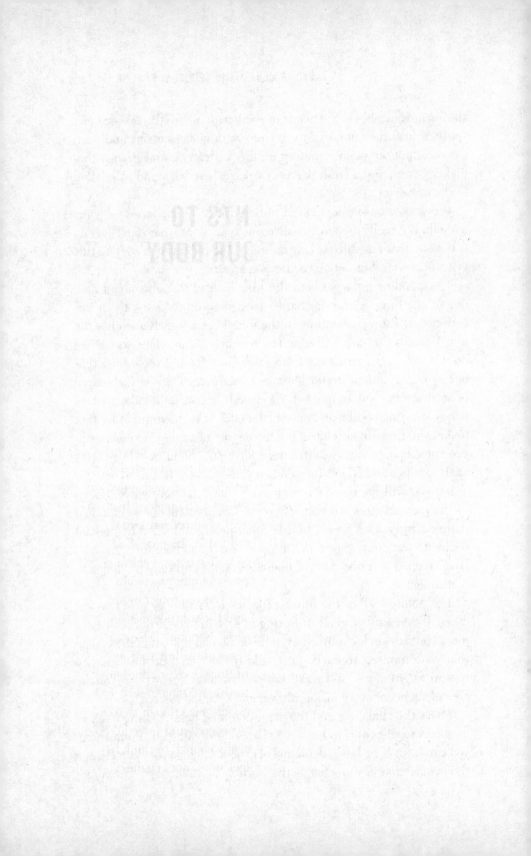

8

SUPPLEMENTS TO FINE-TUNE YOUR BODY

During my vision quest I was living like a modern-day caveman—if only for four days—so I decided to pull myself together and act like one. The nighttime mountain lion visit that happened only in my head still spooked me. All of my senses were on high alert. Instead of waiting for real mountain lions to eat me, I ventured out into the cool night and piled brush at the entrance to First Woman cave, knowing that some indigenous cultures have used such a natural alarm system to keep wild animals at bay. My little pocket knife practically wilted in my hand when I realized how useless it was to protect myself.

To be fair, it wasn't *entirely* the fast and the solitude messing with my head. There truly are predators in the Sonoran Desert, and in principle, some of them are powerful enough to kill you and leave your corpse for crows and turkey buzzards to pick clean. But I grew up backpacking in remote places similar to this Arizona desert; I knew that none of the animals around there were big enough that they'd tangle with a human unless they were cornered and forced to fight. There's not going to be a mountain lion silly enough to think that I'm suitable prey, and the bears are little black ones, not grizzlies.

But your fear doesn't care what you *know*. It thrives on what you *feel*, and it can use your feelings to overwhelm your rational brain. Even though the vast majority of us no longer have to fear animal predators (seriously, when was the last time you worried about being eaten?), we still have to deal with the imprint that our ancestral fears have left inside us. The evolutionary imprint is what makes us so susceptible to cravings: the fear that we won't have enough food or companionship or other comforts. My sense of impending starvation and my delusion that mountain lions were about to attack me came from the exact same place. In today's world of plenty, the disconnect between our primal fears and the endless modern indulgences being pushed toward us can put us into a profoundly dysfunctional state.

Fortunately, that evolutionary legacy also gifted us with a powerful set of tools for conquering those cravings and tapping into the strengths that enabled our ancestors to survive—all of our ancestors, going back to the very first cell on Earth some 3.8 billion years ago. Over the days when I was fasting inside the cave, I slowly became aware of those powers inside me. And there's nothing special about me. Intermittent fasting, multiday fasting, sleep hygiene, exercise, controlled breathing, and spiritual exploration will give every reader of this book—including you—the ability to summon the same powers. Add the right biohacks, and you can crank your powers even higher.

There are a time and a place for biohacks, things that give you an advantage biologically so you will get more of the effects you want more quickly. I could have hooked a little monitor up to my earlobe, which would have helped me use subtle variations in my heart rate to exit the fight-or-flight mode. I could have turned off my hunger with MCT oil. I could have taken brain-boosting nootropic compounds to sharpen my rational thinking or plant medicines to make the cave melt into insignificance. But I wouldn't have realized my particular, transformative vision quest if I hadn't pushed through the day on my own. Don't let your ego trick you into leaning on biohacks to distract you from learning the lessons you may be seeking on a spiritual fast. Sometimes the best way *out* is *through*.

Pushing through is exactly what I worked on that night. I closed my eyes and finally fell asleep as the fire at the cave entrance died down.

By then, something was definitely changing inside me. I was buzzing with energy even as my eyelids drooped shut.

Two hours later, in the middle of the night, a loud rustling noise abruptly woke me from my deep slumber. This time, the noise was very real, not something conjured up by my lizard brain.

THE CHEMICAL EQUATION OF YOU

Fasting is a spiritual process. Fasting is a chemical process. There is no contradiction between these two ideas. They are both valid and equally true.

Whether or not you consider yourself a spiritual person, intermittent fasting will shift your mood and your perceptions in ways that will enable you to look at your life differently. Those mood and perceptual shifts are the result of chemical processes in your body, but they are not chemical *experiences.* You could say the same about pain and fear or about love and pleasure. An experience is something that arises out of your conscious existence, and consciousness arises out of the chemistry of your brain—but nobody knows how that happens. Your molecules and your mind live side by side inside your head. How the two are connected is perhaps the greatest mystery in all of science.

David Chalmers, a philosopher at New York University, summed up the absurd situation in an influential paper titled "Facing Up to the Problem of Consciousness." In it, he wrote, "It is widely agreed that experience arises from a physical basis, but we have no good explanation of why and how it so arises. Why should physical processing give rise to a rich inner life at all? It seems objectively unreasonable that it should, and yet it does."[1]

Fortunately, we don't need to understand exactly *how* we think in order to do it. Humans have been thinking quite effectively for the past 300,000 years without having a theory of consciousness. Likewise, we don't have to understand every detail of the relationship between molecules and mind to know that one affects the other—and that intermittent fasting can do wonders for both. Fasting improves your focus and slows the aging process. It promotes autophagy and detoxification, helping your cells get rid of their built-up waste. And yes, it opens the path to great spiritual journeys, if you want to go there.

All through this book, you've learned about various biohacks that make fasting less painful, more pleasurable, and above all more enriching. A lot of them involve being disciplined about what and when you eat. But we can get even more detailed and targeted than that. To get the most out of your diet—to give the most effective kick to both your molecules and your mind—you will want to make sure that your body has the right supply of the stuff it needs to repair itself, things such as vitamins, minerals, amino acids, and other vital compounds. That is: you will want to take supplements.

At this point, there are several questions people usually ask. The first is some variation of "Why do I need supplements if I eat a balanced diet? I get my nutrients from food, just like our ancestors did." The answer to that is simply that if you are planning to get your nutrients from only what you eat, it will work, as long as you also get toxins only from Mother Nature. And of course, that's not possible. The reality is that the environment we live in is full of thousands of synthetic chemicals and stressors that we did not evolve to handle, along with natural chemicals that are processed and concentrated by Big Food in novel ways, not to mention global diseases such as COVID-19 that can travel more quickly than ever before. Your body needs more nutrients than you can get from food alone to handle that toxin load.

There is also the question of whether food really has the same nutrients it used to, and the answer is a resounding "no!" That's because we have depleted our soil by growing monoculture plant crops without rotating grazing animals, by spraying crops with glyphosate (an herbicide used to kill weeds), and by using industrial farming practices. There are countless studies comparing the nutrient level of modern foods to their levels fifty years ago, which have shown that overall, food—even organic food—is not as nutritious as it used to be. The final reason is even more apocalyptic than losing our soil: it's the rising level of carbon dioxide, or CO_2, in the air. We all learn in elementary school that animals breathe oxygen, and plants breathe CO_2. What happens when plants have a lot more CO_2? They grow more quickly, which means they get bigger, but they have less time to concentrate minerals from the soil. This transformation is already affecting food quality.[2]

You are also likely to need supplements to balance out the effects of fasting. If you're doing intermittent fasting, you may be consuming the exact same number of calories you normally do and getting the same amount of nutrients you usually do. But what if you actually eat fewer calories because you're less hungry? What if you fast for longer periods? If you eat less food, you will get fewer nutrients—that's just simple math.

People also ask, "Will I still get the full benefits of supplements if I take them while I'm fasting? And won't taking those supplements effectively end my fast?" There are no black-and-white answers here, but there are reasonable answers based on what we think we know about how the body works. Whether or not you ought to take a specific supplement during your fast depends on what it is and on how your body normally responds to it when you are not fasting. For example, some vitamins have to be taken with food. Usually, that's either because the vitamin is fat soluble (the body is better able to absorb it when fat is also present), or it's because you'll feel sick if you take it on an empty stomach.

There are two good strategies here for the "take with food" supplements. One is to simply stop taking them, which works fine. You probably won't die if you miss a few days of supplements, so you can go on a "supplement fast" along with avoiding food. Regardless of whether you're fasting or not, there's a case for occasionally mixing up or skipping what you take. It's that you don't want your body to get metabolically lazy by downregulating its own production of protective compounds; this is another example of how the body hates constancy. The other strategy is to do what I do: take some supplements that require food even when I'm when fasting, knowing I'll still absorb some of the compounds. The problem is that no supplement company on Earth writes "Take with food or you will barf" on the label, so it's hard to know *why* it says to take a supplement with food.

It's quite easy to figure this out—take a few of your supplements on an empty stomach. If you feel as though they're going to come back up, *break your fast right away*, which will stop the nausea. There, now you know which supplements *not* to take on an empty stomach. There are some guidelines for you below. No one wants to taste vitamins a second time.

Making things more complicated, some supplements have additive effects when they're taken together, such as vitamins A, D, and K_2. You can take vitamin K_2 any time of day. Vitamin D is best taken in the morning, or at least before noon, because it is a circadian hormone that helps to wake you up, and with a meal, because it is fat soluble. Vitamin A is best taken with meals because it is fat soluble. You see how this goes: if you are dosing up on all three vitamins together, you'll get the biggest bang for your buck by taking them in the morning with a meal.

But wait; most people who read this book and try intermittent fasting will be skipping breakfast most of the time, just because they feel a lot better doing so. How are you going to take your morning fat-soluble vitamins D, A, and K_2? Especially while there's a novel coronavirus running amok, you must manage your vitamin D levels. This combination of nutrients powerfully supports your immune system, bones, and cardiovascular system. Your best bet is to take them on an empty stomach, knowing that they may not absorb as well but *will still absorb*. You could also take them when you break your daily fast. Since I have Bulletproof Coffee most mornings, with enough fat in it to stimulate nutrient absorption, I take my supplements with it. On mornings when I have black coffee, I take them, too—and I have quickly learned which ones you really don't want to take on an empty stomach. After a little while, you will learn to fine-tune your fasts, figuring out which eating rhythms, foods, and supplements work best for you.

BEWARE OF THE BARFY FOUR

Some supplements will reliably ruin a fast. Not because they'll change your metabolism but because of what they do to you on an empty stomach. I call them the "Barfy Four." Do I need to say more?

The first of the Barfy Four supplements to watch out for during fasting is the B vitamins. If you want to experience the worst ever day of fasting, start out with a B complex on an empty stomach. If you can keep it down, you'll taste it all day and wish you hadn't, but most people get nausea from it. Steer clear of B complex. However, vitamin B12 is an important supplement, and the lozenges or capsules don't cause nausea in most people.

The second way is multivitamins. All-in-one pills often contain low-quality formulations of vitamins, and they contain B complex. To top things off, multivitamin pills are typically manufactured with fillers and additives that are difficult for the body to absorb, so you may not even get the benefits of the active ingredients. To be honest, avoiding multivitamins is good advice in general. You simply can't fit a meaningful dose of a useful number of vitamins or minerals into one or two capsules, and what you get is sometimes worse than nothing at all. That certainly is true during a fast.

The third is fish oil. This is a marvelous supplement, and you can take this one with Bulletproof Coffee. If you take it with black coffee or an empty stomach, though, you'll probably feel nauseated. Plus, you will taste it all day. Pro tip: if you get nasty fish burps from your fish oil, it is likely rancid. Go for a great brand that doesn't have a strong flavor.

Finally, you can count on iron supplements and multimineral supplements to cause nausea, acid reflux, or both. Most people can handle single minerals, such as magnesium or zinc, without a problem on an empty stomach. Bundle a bunch of them together, and it's a different story.

When considering how to approach supplements during a fast, it's important to consider the reason you're fasting to begin with. If you are fasting for weight loss or energy or spiritual reasons, you can do what you want. But if you're looking to allow your gut to rest and heal, avoid most if not all supplements. Even if they are formulated well, multivitamins disrupt a gut-rest fast. You should also avoid prebiotic fiber and C8 MCT oil during a gut rest fast. You'll still want to make sure you're consuming some electrolyte minerals, including magnesium, potassium, and sodium. If you're working with a functional medicine physician on gut healing, you'll probably have some herbs to take, too.

As for the question of whether you're cheating on your fast if you take supplements, the dogmatic fasting purists will tell you that anything other than water breaks a fast. In this case, they simply do not understand the true meaning of fasting, *going without*. You can have Bulletproof Coffee without breaking your fast if you're fasting for metabolic reasons, antiaging reasons, or energy. I believe that you can take supplements, too. You're still in *going without* mode. That said, be aware that some supplements, especially drink mixes, contain sugar. During a fast, you want to limit yourself strictly—no more than 20 calories a day from sugar and ideally none.

There are a couple things that you absolutely must avoid during a fast. One is proton pump inhibitors—these drugs block stomach acid production, and you'll probably have a hard time digesting food at the end of a fast if you block this important digestive function with drugs. If it is a prescription, ask your doctor about skipping a day or three. Another thing you must avoid is food additives: artificial colorings, flavorings, MSG, and sweeteners. They wreck your gut bacteria and often cause intense cravings.

Here's the bottom line. In general, you can take vitamin and mineral supplements during an intermittent fast and still get full fat-burning benefits. You have to be more restrictive if you want to do a gut rest as well. And you should be informed about the specific effects of the supplements you're taking, because some of them can affect your body's function during your fast. For instance, they can:

- Decrease your blood sugar, possibly zapping your energy and giving you brain fog

- Raise your glucose level, taking you out of ketosis (the whole point of fasting)

- Pass through your body without as much being absorbed as when they are taken with food

- Make you nauseated if you take them on an empty stomach

Taking vitamins and supplements while doing intermittent fasting requires some experimentation. When you fast, you will probably experience more sensitivity to your supplements. It's possible that you will get really tired or will experience intense hunger and cravings after you take your supplements—if so, they're probably not working for you. Time to mix things up.

To be honest, every aspect of fasting requires you to be aware of your state. Being Bulletproof is all about paying attention to how your body feels and adjusting accordingly. To help you out, I've broken down some of the major classes of supplements that you should consider and summarized their effects.

THE SUPPLEMENT CHECKLIST

ACTIVATED CHARCOAL

This is the number one supplement I suggest taking during a fast, yet most people overlook it. It isn't sexy, I guess. Activated charcoal is a black powder made of coconut shells, peat, sawdust, olive pits, or bone char. (The charcoal I designed for Bulletproof uses only coconut and is the finest-size particle to maximize effectiveness.) It is heated to extremely high temperatures, which makes it more porous than regular charcoal. It's quite different from the briquettes you use on your barbecue. Activated charcoal has a huge surface area—1 teaspoon of it has a surface area the size of a soccer field!—and a negative electrical charge that draws positively charged toxins toward it. It traps toxins and chemicals in your gut, preventing them from being absorbed into your bloodstream. Instead of these poisons becoming a part of whatever fat you're carrying around, they leave your body as waste products.

Getting rid of the toxins floating in your body will slow the aging process and help you think more clearly. Fasting alone will give you a detox, but activated charcoal will help. In fact, studies show that activated charcoal extends life span even if you aren't fasting. It also absorbs stress-producing chemicals produced by bacteria in your gut, reduces cholesterol, and promotes kidney function. Here's one more really cool thing about activated charcoal: it will reduce the severity of your cravings during your fast. It's startling: you get cravings, you take charcoal, and now you don't feel hungry anymore. What's going on? The bacteria in your gut are freaking out because they don't have any food, either, which causes them to produce lipopolysaccharides and various toxins that give you physical stress. You interpret that response as emotional stress, which in turn can trigger cravings and irritability. Activated charcoal cuts that cycle off at the foundation, so you can happily go about your fast.

A small downside is that activated charcoal can make you a little bit constipated. That's not going to be a major problem during fasting, since you're not moving food through your body anyway. It also absorbs any medication you take at the same time, so be careful.

Daily dose: 1 to 10 1,000 mg capsules, away from medications, fewer if you get constipated. Any time of day or night.

SYSTEMIC PROTEOLYTIC ENZYMES

Your body makes enzymes to speed its biochemical reactions. Proteolytic enzymes break down proteins; you use them when you eat protein. But systemic enzymes are not enzymes that are meant to act on your steak; they're meant to act on *you*. If you're trying to crank up your body's self-cleaning autophagy, take these enzymes. They are normally produced in the pancreas, but if you take them as supplements, you can boost your enzyme levels and give your pancreas a rest. Proteolytic enzymes break down unneeded proteins in the body as part of the general process of flushing out cellular junk. The two most popular forms of these enzymes are serrapeptase and nattokinase. Serrapeptase is made by silkworms, which use the enzyme to dissolve their cocoons after metamorphosis (that's how we discovered it!). Thankfully, now it's made by fermentation. Nattokinase is derived from fermented soybeans, a particularly unappetizing, slimy, nutty dish you might find at a Japanese restaurant called *natto*. Proteolytic enzymes are great for cardiovascular health. They also help break up clotting factors (which can cause dangerous blood clots) and scar tissue in the body, as well as remove worn-out immune molecules from your blood.

There are also animal-based systemic proteolytic enzymes. For me, these are the gold standard, because they are broader spectrum than the plant-based ones. There are several different brands of proteolytic enzymes that aid digestion. Wobenzym is a good one. If you're going to be fasting and you're saving money by not eating, you might as well splurge on proteolytic enzymes. They promote optimal nutrient digestion and absorption, which are key to gut health. They tell your body, "Hey, you got everything you need. Just go work on yourself. Fold some proteins. Get rid of some dead stuff. Do your job."

You feel better. Your blood flow improves. It's a good move. I therefore tend to take a very high dose of proteolytic enzymes when I am fasting. When I was recovering from being obese, I sometimes took one hundred capsules a day on an empty stomach; they are considered safe, but the normal dose is 1 to 4 capsules. I have been taking at least 10 high-dose (120,000 SPU each) serrapeptase supplements while fasting for ten years, along with six animal-based proteolytic enzymes. They are a waste of money to take if you have food in yours stomach.

Daily dose: 1 to 2 120,000 SU serrapeptase capsules and/or 1 to 2 2000 FU nattokinase capsules; 1 to 2 proteolytic enzyme capsules such as Wobenzym or BiOptimizers Masszymes.

ADAPTOGENS AND MUSHROOMS

These can help you power through stress responses. Adaptogens are powerful herbs that originated in China and Russia. They were originally used by the military because of their ability to help manage the body's stress response. They make it easy for you to turn on your stress response and then easy for you to turn it off when you don't need it anymore. Otherwise, once your stress response is turned on, it tends to stay on for long periods of time. This was an advantage for soldiers who needed to be able to run into combat and then rest afterward. You're probably not going into combat, but you do experience stress. The ability to turn your stress response on and off quickly is something that can help you live longer. It can help you fast, too.

It's not uncommon to get hypoglycemia when you start fasting, especially when you don't yet have ketones present (either from natural ketosis or from MCT oil). If this is your first time fasting—and especially if you didn't ramp up slowly from just skipping breakfast but instead jumped right in and attempted a weekend fast and exercise at the same time—it's going to be a bit tough. You're probably going to get slightly dizzy. You might experience brain fog and headaches; you might get supercranky; you might start sleeping less. It might seem as though your spouse or partner has suddenly turned into a total jerk. In fact, if you notice that everyone around you has suddenly become stupid, it's a pretty good sign that your blood sugar is low.

These feelings will go away once you teach your metabolism to behave itself. By far the easiest way to do this is to start your first few fasts with Bulletproof Coffee. I'm not saying this to get you to buy Bulletproof Coffee—people have had about 200 million cups of Bulletproof Coffee so far, and the company is doing just fine, thank you. I'm saying it because it will make your entry into fasting painless, and I don't like pain unless it serves a purpose.

The other way to make your fasts less painful and more effective is to allow your body to produce cortisol when it needs to raise your blood sugar and then to stop producing it when your blood sugar returns to normal. This is a function of your adrenal glands, and it is totally normal. Adaptogenic herbs make that process work better. The main adaptogenic herbs are ashwagandha, rhodiola, holy basil, ginseng, and the mushrooms cordyceps, reishi, and lion's mane. Ashwagandha and rhodiola are classic stress-modulating adaptogens. Holy basil and ginseng are also anti-inflammatory, as are adaptogenic cordyceps. Reishi is particularly relaxing; lion's mane aids nerve regeneration. I've had my best results with the Australian species of these mushrooms, but you should experiment to see what works best for you.

If you're a masochist, you can make adaptogen or mushroom tea or coffee. Expect a bitter, earthy flavor. But there's no reason to choke down mushroom tea; you can take adaptogenic mushrooms as capsules or liquid droppersful. Powdered mushrooms are not as strong as a high-quality extract, and I've never experienced any benefit from taking them in that form. There's a reason for that: some compounds in mushrooms can be extracted only with hot water, others only by alcohol. If you're going to all the trouble of buying adaptogen mushrooms, I would highly encourage you to go for the liquid extracts. Pro tip: putting mushroom powder into your coffee is a terrible idea because it tastes nasty, and there's no benefit to polluting the taste of your coffee anyway. The best mushroom extracts are dual-extracted with alcohol and hot water, then bottled in glass bottles with droppers. The flavor is mild (you can put it into your coffee without ruining it) and the effect is dramatic.

Daily dose: Adaptogens come in different strengths of extraction and in different combinations, so follow what the label says. Most companies suggest the smallest dose because of labeling requirements. I usually find that I do well by adding 50 percent to the label dose. You should experiment to see what works best for you.

STRESSORS

You also might want to increase the stress on your body during your fast. Sounds weird, I know—I was just telling you how to decrease stress with adaptogens. That is adrenal stress. Oxidative stress is another type of stress that comes from your metabolism. You can do some very good things to your biology if you mildly stress your cells in a precise way to promote autophagy and to create better cellular antioxidant response. The simple way to do that is to cut back on some of the antioxidant supplements you might already be taking, especially coenzyme Q10 and vitamin C. Doing so will allow more oxidative stress, which will create a response that helps your cells become better at manufacturing their own on-board antioxidants, which then can bump up your rate of autophagy. What's happening is that your body is saying, "Oh, man, I'm really struggling here. I'm going to break down those old parts of the cells to have energy for making new cells." It's a way of prompting your body to switch into renewal mode. I usually take these supplements as I'm ending an intermittent fast (normally, I have them with dinner).

Daily dose: My dosing advice for stressors mirrors my advice for vitamins and minerals, below.

WATER-SOLUBLE VITAMINS

Everyone knows the value of taking vitamins. It's right there in the name: "vitamin" is a contraction of "vital amines," a name given to them by the Polish chemist Casimir Funk in 1912. Funk discovered a group of chemicals called amines that he determined were essential for human health. Today, we know that not all vitamins fit into that one chemical family, but he got the idea right—you really do need these compounds. To get the most out of them, you need to know what the various vitamins do, how much of them you need, and—especially if you are fasting—when to take them.

You can process water-soluble vitamins just fine even if you haven't eaten in a while. Actually, you'll get the most benefit from taking these vitamins and supplements on an empty stomach, because they are best absorbed that way. Spread them out during your fasting period to reduce the potential for stomach upset. Then if one of them makes you feel sick, you can easily pinpoint the culprit.

Daily dose: For vitamins and minerals, I recommend taking twice as much as the recommended daily allowance (RDA), unless your lab tests show that you need a lot more or that you have too much of something. Vitamin C requires much higher doses. I take 2 grams per day unless I'm sick or stressed, in which case I take even more.

- **B vitamins and folate (also known as vitamin B9):** You can take B vitamins during a fasting period, though as I warned you earlier, taking them on an empty stomach could make you feel nauseated. If that happens to you, try taking B vitamins after a cup of Bulletproof Coffee (the quality fats may help prevent stomach upset). Or just take these vitamins when you break your fast. Vitamin B_{12} can protect against dementia, increase immune function, maintain nerves, and regenerate cells. It also protects you from atherosclerosis and maintains the chemical reactions that repair DNA and prevent cancer. One of the most crucial areas in which B_{12} operates is the brain. Folate and B_{12} are both required for optimal mental function; a deficiency in one produces a deficiency in the other, but folate will not correct a B_{12} deficiency in the brain. Folate also supports a healthy heart and nervous system. Beware: if you make the mistake of treating B_{12} deficiency without folate, you can potentially suffer permanent brain damage. Likewise, taking high amounts of folate without also getting adequate B_{12} can cause neurological conditions. To be safe, I always take them together. For most people, methylcobalamin and hydroxycobalamin are the best forms of B_{12}, and folate is superior to folic acid.

- **Vitamin C:** Like the B vitamins, you can take vitamin C with water during a fasting period. It is usually easy on an empty stomach if you don't have reflux, and overall it is one of the safest, most effective supplements you can take. Vitamin C is needed for collagen and connective tissue formation. It's used to manufacture glutathione, one of the most powerful antioxidants in the body. Studies indicate that vitamin C can enhance your immune system and can help quench the aging-related molecular fragments known as free radicals. Even quite high doses are safe. When you're fasting, 500 milligrams to 1 gram twice a day is a good idea for basic support. If you are doing more intensive healing or battling a virus or infection, the protocol for vitamin C is to take increasing doses of it until you get loose stools, then back off a little bit. When you're sick, your body can oftentimes absorb 20 or 30 grams orally before you hit that limit. When you are well, the limit might be 3 or 4 grams. A startling 30 percent of Americans are deficient in vitamin C.[3] I am ambivalent about vitamin C when I fast and take it sometimes and not others. It lasts in the body for only about eight hours, so divided doses are better.

FAT-SOLUBLE VITAMINS

Vitamin A, D, E, and K dissolve in fat, not in water, so it's best to take them during your eating window. If you're doing Bulletproof Intermittent Fasting, you can take fat-soluble vitamins with your Bulletproof Coffee, which contains fats such as grass-fed butter and Brain Octane C8 MCT oil. Since I have that most mornings during my fast, I take vitamins A, D, and K at the same time.

- **Vitamin A** supports the proper functioning of the heart, lungs, kidneys, and immune system. You want that, right? But a quarter of Americans consume less than half the recommended daily allowance (RDA) of vitamin A, which is already set too low by the US Food and Drug Administration. Many people mistakenly believe that they can get vitamin A from eating plants, especially carrots. Sorry, Bugs Bunny, but that's not how it works. Plants don't contain vitamin A; they contain beta-carotene, and the body is not very good at converting beta-carotene into vitamin A. The result is that some people develop vitamin A deficiency even while consuming far more beta-carotene than they require. Unless you eat a lot of liver or oysters, taking real, preformed vitamin A is a good idea, whether you are fasting or not. It can improve your immunity and even your sleep. I prefer 10,000 IU per day. It's okay to take it when most convenient for you, but bedtime is the ideal time.

- **Vitamin D** is a superbiohack that fights the aging process and enhances performance. It facilitates the movement of hormones around the body and adjusts the action of more than one thousand genes. It moderates immune function and inflammation and aids in calcium metabolism and bone formation. I'm a fan: I found that I got sick far less often once I began taking vitamin D supplements, and there are now hundreds of scientific studies showing that it makes you more metabolically resilient. Your body can make this vitamin on its own from sunlight and cholesterol, but unless you live near the equator or run around without any clothes most of the time, you probably aren't making enough of it. This is one of the supplements you ought to be taking most of the time for the rest of your life unless a blood test says you have high levels. It's even more important if your skin is dark. Take this one in the morning. Because blood levels vary widely when people take the same amount of D_3, it's best to get a blood test to ensure your vitamin D_3 levels are between 60 and 90 ng/ml. An average person will require about 1,000 IU of vitamin D_3 for every 25 pounds of body weight, although blood tests showed me that I require twice that amount. Get tested, seriously!

- **Vitamin E** protects the fats in your cell membranes from destructive oxidation. It plays an important role in protecting your skin from damage and aging caused by the troublesome free radicals (charged molecules) that form when you're exposed to the ultraviolet rays of the sun. There are eight forms of vitamin E, and you want a supplement that has mixed tocopherols and tocotrienols and the gamma and delta forms. Avoid synthetic vitamin E; it is bad for you. If you have been vegan, you'll require a lot more vitamin E than normal to repair your cells. For most people, 400 IU per day with other fats in any meal or beverage is enough.

- **Vitamin K** is a stealth nutrient. People think they can get it from eating vegetables, but there are two types of vitamin K: K_1 and K_2. Unless you grew up eating only grass-fed meat and raw milk, you're probably deficient in vitamin K_2. It is a fat-soluble vitamin that helps with calcium metabolism. When it isn't processed properly by your body, excess calcium is deposited in your arteries, leading to calcification and stiffening. This is why vitamin K_2 helps prevent atherosclerosis and heart attacks while strengthening your bones. Since vitamin D helps metabolize calcium, vitamins D and K_2 work together synergistically. There are two forms that matter, called MK-4 and MK-7. Take your K_2 with vitamin D_3 in the morning. In the formulation I put together for Bulletproof, I included 1500 mg of MK-4 and 300 mcg of MK-7. It is safe to take higher doses of K$_2$ if you have calcification problems, however.

MINERALS

These are also highly recommended during a fast, with a caveat: it is possible that taking large amounts of zinc, chromium, or vanadium while fasting can drop your blood sugar level even more than normal. If you find that you're hitting really low blood sugar levels after taking minerals, you might need to make adjustments.

- **Iodine:** For maximum absorption, take kelp powder or potassium iodide capsules with food. Pass on iodized table salt: common iodized table salt is mixed with anticaking agents and other unwanted compounds and is chemically bleached. Iodine is very helpful for keeping your thyroid working well while you're fasting. It also enhances immune function, prevents brain damage, and overall helps maintain a healthy metabolism. Iodine deficiency is widespread, so taking a supplement is a good idea. Physically active people are at especially high risk of iodine deficiency because they lose iodine through sweat. Supplement ranges vary widely, from 150 mcg in kelp, all the way up to several milligrams per day. Take it in the morning.

- **Magnesium:** When beginning a magnesium supplement routine, some people report getting what you might delicately call "disaster pants" (loose stool or worse). If you have a sensitive stomach, you should seriously consider taking your magnesium with food! That will reduce the likelihood of negative effects. If you're taking magnesium to help you sleep, take it after your last meal of the day. However, since your body level of magnesium is at its highest at noon, I take half of mine in the morning and half at bedtime. The body uses magnesium in more than three hundred different enzymatic processes, including all of those

involved in ATP (energy) production in your mitochondria.
Magnesium is also vital for proper transcription of DNA and
RNA—an essential process every time your body creates a new
cell. Almost all Americans are deficient in magnesium. The
majority don't consume the RDA, and many studies show that
the RDA levels are already set too low.[4] Due to soil depletion
and overintensive modern farming practices, it's almost
impossible to get enough magnesium from your regular diet.
Without a doubt, everyone should supplement with magnesium.
Take at least 800 mg per day, and up to 2 grams if it doesn't
cause disaster pants. (Magnesium has a laxative effect.)

- **Potassium and sodium:** Both potassium and sodium (which
  you get from good old-fashioned sea salt) are important
  supplements, doing jobs that complement the work of
  magnesium in your body. When your mitochondria are working
  on restoring themselves, they need magnesium and potassium.
  They rely on these minerals whether they're stressed or not, but
  the need is more acute when they're stressed. You can't get one
  of these minerals into your cells without the other. You therefore
  want to take magnesium and potassium together when you're
  fasting. Don't overdo potassium, because a very small percentage
  of people get heart arrhythmias from potassium overdoses. Your
  body requires a couple grams per day from all sources, and many
  people are deficient. You can get potassium in powdered form as
  potassium bicarbonate, which is similar to baking soda. It works
  really well. Most people can handle a couple hundred milligrams
  daily. When you're fasting, if you're drinking only water and also
  if you're in ketosis, you need even more of these minerals. Take
  some sea salt for sodium as well, so that your potassium and
  sodium don't get out of balance. Just don't be stupid and chow
  down on lots of potassium powder, because it can dysregulate
  the electrical flow in your body. A lot of people do very well by
  taking regular sodium bicarbonate. It is literally baking soda! It
  increases the alkalinity of the body, which is beneficial to your
  mitochondria. Personally, I take both potassium bicarbonate and

a little bit of sodium bicarbonate, which aids in antiaging and longevity. Take them before bed, at least 200 mg, but at doses safe for your own risk factors.

- **Chromium and vanadium:** These minerals modulate your insulin levels and can improve your weight loss during fasting. If you overdo it, though, they can drop your blood sugar level too low. If your insulin levels dip, you run the risk of hypoglycemia, or low blood sugar. Even a small bout of hypoglycemia can lead to problems adjusting and managing your moods. Take these supplements when you break your fast. I prefer 200 to 400 mg of chromium polynicotinate with 2 mg of vanadyl sulfate.

- **Zinc and copper:** These two minerals work better together, so you'll often see them combined in pill form. They perform hundreds of critical health tasks. Combined, they can form a powerful antioxidant called copper-zinc superoxide dismutase, or CuZnSOD. It is one of your body's most potent natural defense mechanisms against aging and molecular damage. Zinc is a key mineral in the support of healthy immune function, energy production, and mood. It can be tough to get enough from food, and your body doesn't store it, meaning you need to replenish it each day. You need copper to work in conjunction with zinc and for proper vascular and heart function. I take them together, because too much zinc can decrease the copper level in your body. The best form I have found is zinc and copper orotate, which is used in the formula I created for Bulletproof: 15 mg zinc orotate and 2 mg copper orotate, taken with food.

OTHER SUPPLEMENTS

There is a world of other supplements you can take while fasting, including amino acids, oils, and various herbs and herbal extracts. (Some of the adaptogens I mentioned earlier fall into the last category.) You can experiment to see which ones work for you and at what doses and timing.

- **L-tyrosine** is an amino acid that should to be taken on an empty stomach. It boosts mood and cognition, enhances your physical and mental stress response, and encourages healthy glandular function. It quickly crosses the blood-brain barrier to boost the neurotransmitters (brain-signaling chemicals) dopamine, epinephrine, and norepinephrine. It's also a building block of thyroid hormone, and having more thyroid hormone available during a fast makes you feel good. Your body can make it, but it depletes when you're stressed. In the modern lifestyle, most people's natural production can't keep up with the demand. Studies have shown that cadets in combat training supplementing with L-tyrosine had reduced negative effects from physical and psychosocial stress on mental performance. Try 750 mg to 1,500 mg in the morning before eating any protein.

- **L-glutamine** is another effective amino acid, good for healing the gut. Together with related branched-chain amino acids, or BCAAs, these supplements are usually a no-go while fasting because they will throw you out of ketosis faster than anyone's business by raising your insulin levels. If you feel as though you're dying during your fast and just really dragging—or maybe you are having terrible headaches—you can take some L-glutamine for relief. It's going to turn your brain on in about five minutes, but you won't have the benefits of ketosis that you get from an extended fast. You'll still be fasting, but this is not an ideal strategy. At least you will still get some of the other benefits of fasting. You are better off taking BCAA and L-glutamine between meals on days when you're not fasting or at the end of a fast. They work best on an empty stomach. If you really want to take these supplements during a fast while staying in ketosis, combine them with Brain Octane MCT oil, which supplies your body with extra ketones. For regular use, 2 to 4 grams per day is plenty, taken on an empty stomach.

- **Fish oil and krill oil:** This is a tricky one. Small doses of high-quality fish oil reduce inflammation, improve brain function, boost mood, suppress anxiety and depression, enhance muscle growth, and even work as a sleep aid. But poor-quality fish oil or long-term high doses can cause more problems than they solve. You also need to be choosy, because not all fish oil is created equal. Most of the brands you are likely to find at your local supermarket or your corner drugstore are contaminated, oxidized, and generally not very potent. If you cannot find a high-quality fish oil, you are better off avoiding it altogether. I recommend a combination of fish oil, krill oil, and fish egg oil. Krill oil is harder to find, but it is more stable and it has a chemical formulation that makes it easier for your brain to use. It also contains astaxanthin, a so-called keto-carotenoid that is a potent antioxidant molecule. Oil supplements are easier for your body to absorb if they're taken with food. You should take them during your eating window or with your Bulletproof Coffee, 1 to 2 grams per day.

- **Ginger and turmeric:** These roots come straight from nature's medicine chest. Ginger attacks inflammation through the action of compounds known as gingerols, shogaols, and paradols. Ginger is also a natural pain reliever, chemically related to ibuprofen, good for treating arthritis and joint discomfort. Turmeric has been a staple of Ayurvedic medicine for thousands of years. Its primary active ingredient is curcumin, the chemical that gives it the distinctive yellow color. Curcumin is a potent antioxidant that has been clinically documented to reduce inflammation, inhibit the growth of tumor cells, and improve insulin resistance. In addition, scientists have discovered that turmeric contains some two dozen anti-inflammatory compounds. And since I'm both a biohacker and a chef, I love the flavor of ginger and turmeric. You can take them both while you're fasting, though they can be a little bit spicy on an empty stomach. Dose varies so widely based on the brand you choose that it's hard to recommend it here. In my formula for

Bulletproof, I combine 500 mg of turmeric extract with other herbs. However, if you were eating plain turmeric or using a plain powder, you'd require a lot more than 500 mg.

- **Antimicrobials and probiotics** work to establish a harmonious relationship between you and the ecosystem of bacteria living inside you. Any herbs that you're taking for their antimicrobial or antiyeast properties are particularly useful while you're fasting. I use grapefruit seed extract, a natural broad-spectrum antimicrobial, to help fix my gut during fasting, It makes a big difference. Probiotics build up the population of good bacteria in the gut and are generally a good idea all around. Probiotics work very well during fasting if you use prebiotic fiber to turn off your hunger. (Remember, prebiotics make fasting easy by suppressing hunger, but if you're on a "gut rest" fast where you want nothing in your gut, skip them.) The probiotics will use the prebiotic fiber as fuel to grow. In most cases, taking probiotics on an empty gut is a waste of money because they have nothing to eat so they can multiply in your gut! Take them about an hour before the end of a fast so they will pass through your stomach intact, before your stomach naturally raises its acid level to digest a meal. Use the number of capsules or packets recommended for the brand you choose.

- **Exogenous ketones:** No discussion of supplements would be complete without addressing the idea of giving yourself ketone supplements to regulate your fasting state of ketosis. As I stated earlier, most of these exogenous (created outside the body) ketones are a bad idea. Both ketone salts and ketone esters have serious drawbacks, as described earlier in the book. For long-term use, C8 MCT oil is the only ketone source I recommend.

But wait—don't start dosing up just yet! Before you even consider taking supplements while fasting, you should talk to your doctor about potential interactions between the supplements and any prescription medications you may be on. Supplements have a profoundly good safety record compared to even common over-the-counter pharmaceuticals, but there are still interactions to consider.

Most mineral supplements, including calcium, magnesium, potassium, and zinc, can prevent your body from absorbing pharmaceuticals, and some herbs have contraindications. Also, certain medications have to be taken within specific time frames; taking them on an empty stomach or within a restricted eating window could interfere with their effects. Your pharmacist can help you know if it is safe to take something without food, or you can check online references. You can take most vitamins and medications that say "with food" with a Bulletproof Coffee because the fat helps absorption and you will still be fasting. Even a small amount of fat (1 teaspoon of C8 MCT oil plus 1 teaspoon of grass-fed butter) is often enough.

Supplements to Spice up Your Sex Life

Fasting is about embracing life, not turning away from it. Once you adapt to your fast, you may find that your emotions are more intense and your libido is elevated. That's another aspect of your health that you can enhance with some clever biohacks. The following supplements are effective ways to enhance your sex drive naturally.

Arginine: Improves blood vessel dilation, enhancing an erection.

Ashwagandha: An adaptogenic herb that also improves sexual lubrication in women.

Boron: Increases testosterone in men and boosts resistance to vaginal infections in women.

Cnidium: A Chinese herb that activates the same biochemical pathways as prescription erectile dysfunction drugs do (really!) and also has profound antioxidant properties.

Folate: Increases sperm count, enhancing fertility.

Ginko biloba: Raises nitric oxide levels in blood, promoting stronger erections.

Ginseng: A win-win; it treats erectile dysfunction and heightens libido.

Kava: Improves sex drive in women.

Maca: This root, also known as Peruvian ginseng, can reverse erectile problems caused by antidepressants and low desire. Do not consume raw maca, however; it must be gelatinized to work.

Magnesium: Important in reducing stress and calming the mood in the bedroom.

Selenium: Found in the testes; increases male health and fertility.

Turmeric: Balances testosterone levels in men and estrogen levels in women.

Vitamin C: A necessary nutrient for creating sex hormones; also reduces stress.

Vitamin D$_3$: A deficiency of this vitamin is common in men with erectile dysfunction.

Zinc: A key component of oysters; boosts libido and male sexual potency.

9

IT'S A LITTLE DIFFERENT FOR WOMEN

At my makeshift campsite inside First Woman cave—which is regarded as the location where Kamalapukwia, the First Woman of Yavapai mythology, the equivalent of Eve from the Bible, brought forth the ancestors of her tribe and of all the other people on Earth—you could say I was slowly being reborn. It was not exactly going smoothly. I had pushed through the hunger and the imaginary vicious predators, but now I heard a noise coming from inside the cave. A real noise.

I fully expected that my vision quest might cause me to hear voices and to, well, see visions. In fact, I wanted it to happen. This was not what I had bargained for, however. This was no transcendent message of spiritual truths. It was a resolutely physical, menacing, rustling sound. Whatever was causing it was very close to me, somewhere between the cave entrance and my sleeping bag. My rational mind cast around blindly for ideas. My heart was pounding. I growled (seriously, that can scare away many animals, and I have a mean growl) and groped around to find my flashlight. By the time I could turn it on, there was nothing to see.

For the rest of the night, I slept with one eye open, if at all. The noise reoccurred and again; there was nothing to see. When the morning sun finally illuminated the cave entrance, marking my fourth and final day there, I discovered that a little brown bird had been attracted to the pile of brush I'd placed as a protective barrier at the opening of the cave. The bird was nocturnal, and had returned several times during the night with scavenged building materials for building a nest in the brush, making the same rustling noise each time. It seemed hard to believe that I'd been terrified of that harmless little creature, but that's what had happened. I had told myself a story about predators, one I knew was not true, yet I had believed my story, and then I had responded to it emotionally and physically. I had to laugh at my own foolishness. Even after I had faced down my fears by staying alone in the cave, even after I had gained mastery over my hallucinatory mountain lions, my mind had taken advantage of me yet again. It's not easy being reborn, I realized. There's a long process of *becoming* involved in becoming a better, stronger person.

The same is true for my relationship with food. Or your relationship with food—or anyone's relationship with food. Quite possibly you aren't even aware you have a relationship with food, but you most certainly do. It is practically hardwired into us: "I am going to starve if I don't eat in the next few hours." The amygdala, the deep-seated portion of the brain responsible for self-preservation, reacts that way when we deny our body food. Or at least, that's what it does until we teach it not to.

I was determined to continue the process of rebirth that had begun in that cave, even knowing it would probably be long and arduous. Well, of course it would be! Being born the first time is rarely a simple event. Kamalapukwia's birthing was the beginning of the saga of humankind. When we emerge from the womb, it is the beginning of our own unpredictable and meandering path through life. All the things that happened to me in the cave were the beginning of a grand journey, but at least I was on my way. You are on your way, too.

THE OTHER HALF OF THE STORY

There's a huge topic that is inexplicably left out of most discussions about fasting: the way it works for women. In most of the books, articles, news stories, and blog posts about fasting, writers tend to assume that all bodies are identical—or rather, that women are identical to men. In fact, most medical and scientific studies today still use the male body as the test model.[1] A recent review of research papers on intermittent fasting posted in a Harvard database illustrates the situation starkly: only thirteen of the seventy-one studies included women.[2] It's a problematic omission. Sure, we all have the same basic digestive organs, but men and women are not at all biologically the same.

(Quick aside: To keep things simple, I'm going to address "you" in this chapter as if you are a woman. If you are, great. If you aren't, this is a chance to broaden your horizons. Incidentally, nearly equal numbers of men and women read my books based on available data, so it was always a coin flip.)

This is in no way an argument about superiority or inferiority or about strength and weakness. It is purely a matter of biology. In one major for instance, the female body is designed to allow for childbirth and lactation, with all of the physiological specializations that go with them. Men and women have different hormone levels, which means that they respond to diets quite differently. Women between the ages of menarche and menopause have active ovaries and go through menstrual cycles. Women are shorter, on average; they tend to have smaller lungs; they have different distributions of body fat.

Women are also more sensitive to dietary changes at the cellular level. If a woman doesn't have enough energy and nutrients to build a healthy baby, the shortfall very noticeably alters or interrupts her menstrual cycle and will manifest itself in a strong hunger response. Throughout most of history, a starved or malnourished woman had a much higher risk of dying if she became pregnant, much more so than the man who participated in creating the pregnancy. The biological cost of being out of energy is therefore much higher for women—even if they aren't pregnant; even if they are not currently fertile.

For all of these reasons, fasting affects the female body differently than it affects the male body. Because the broad guidelines for fasting have been developed for, and tested on, men, women generally need to do more fine-tuning of their fasts. The good news is that all available evidence suggests that women have just as much to gain from fasting as men do, especially when it comes to disease prevention. Importantly, fasting protects against some of the metabolic causes of Alzheimer's disease, a condition that affects twice as many women as men.

Let's pause for a moment to review the automated systems in a woman's body. Like men, women's bodies are governed by the four F survival rules that drive all higher forms of life: fear, food, er, fertility, and friends. During the years you are fertile, those systems are carefully sensing food, nutrients, and stress levels to determine whether you can achieve that third F. If the number of calories, the type of fat, micronutrients, toxins, or stress are not at acceptable levels, it will trigger physical anxiety, a biological stress response that warns, *The future of our species is at risk!* Men and women are wired at very primitive levels to ensure the creation and survival of the next generation.

When you decide to fast in a way that doesn't overstress your body, it can make you stronger and more metabolically fit. When you fast too much, it can create a stress response more quickly than it would in a man's body. This is based on the fact that nature wants to protect women's bodies as a safe space for gestation. After all, the next generation—and thus the survival of the species—rests on successful pregnancy. Of course, your conscious brain knows that that's all BS. But those ancient survival systems are the same ones that are present in fish and birds, and they are hardwired. It's just Mother Nature protecting your fetus—even though you're not pregnant. She's paranoid that way, apparently. This explains why fasting has a different effect on women than it does on men.

When the amygdala, the primitive lizard part of your brain, believes that your reproductive ability is being compromised, it responds by restricting the secretion of a potent reproductive chemical, gonadotropin-releasing hormone, to preserve resources. Gonadotropin-releasing hormone normally directs the release of two other hormones: follicle-stimulating hormone, which guides sexual maturation and triggers the development of mature eggs, and luteinizing hormone, which prompts the development of a structure called the corpus luteum, ready to implant a fertilized egg in the uterus. But now sex hormone levels are dropping all around. The ovaries respond to this hormonal decline with an act of extreme self-preservation.

The tight connection among food supply, sex hormones, and fertility cycles makes sense from an evolutionary perspective. The pressures of natural selection favored women who were maximally fertile whenever they were healthy enough to reproduce and had access to an adequate supply of food. Even if you're not interested in having a baby, your fertility is an indicator of your overall health. In both women and men, changes in nutrition or caloric intake send environmental signals through the body that can impact the way your genes are expressed. In women, this connection is far more acute, because a woman's body has to invest drastically more energy and resources into creating a baby than a man's has to invest in producing sperm.

The study of the impact of environment on genes is called epigenetics. More and more, biologists are discovering that the ways we live—our lifestyle choices, our environment, our diet—all influence the way our genes are expressed. Epigenetics tells us that our genetic code is not an ironclad, unchanging recipe for who we are. It is instead a menu of options. External influences, which can range from toxins to hunger to chronic stress, flip molecular switches in the body that determine which genes are active and which ones go silent. In other words, your cells are constantly changing the way they read their own DNA. For women, epigenetics helps explain why daily intermittent fasting can pose a challenge. Fasting or eating a low-fat diet instigates epigenetic changes in addition to the chemical changes that tell your body, "There's a famine! Emergency! Don't reproduce!" A male-oriented fasting plan that doesn't take this sensitivity into account could cause serious health compromises—or, more likely, you will simply feel so miserable that you'll give up on fasting too soon.

No wonder, then, that a significant number of women have reported that frequent, ongoing intermittent fasting or repeated longer fasts cause problems including sleeplessness, anxiety, adrenal insufficiency, irregular periods, poor bone health, and even temporary infertility. These reports are backed up by scientific research on laboratory animals.[3] In fact, one rat study showed that two weeks of intermittent fasting shrank ovaries, disrupted sleep, and shut down menstrual cycles in female rats.[4] Intermittent fasting is unlikely to have such drastic effects on you in that amount of time, because Mother Nature knows you're not expected to pump out a large litter of babies every couple months (phew). On the other hand, even without fasting, unending ketosis suppresses menstruation! It is not an appropriate diet for women over long periods of time unless you cycle into and out of it on a regular basis, at which point it is fantastic.

FEMALE FASTING STRATEGIES

Fortunately, women can benefit from fasting without compromising their reproductive health. You just have to make a few smart tweaks. The first is to practice intermittent fasting *every other day*. That way, your body gets the signal that says, "I must be in an area with adequate food for my (nonexistent) baby, but I must be strong enough to go awhile without food." That's the sweet spot. Daily, unending intermittent fasting is too close to a famine for your body, even if you eat enough calories in the evening. It's also important not to work out strenuously on the days you do fast. Go to a yoga class. Do some Pilates. Take a walk. Don't do high-intensity interval training or lift heavy weights on an intermittent fasting day.

Another hack that works for a lot of women is to do Bulletproof Intermittent Fasting with zero carbohydrates and zero protein, just Bulletproof Coffee with grass-fed butter and MCT oil. The many women I've spoken to about this have found that they can fast more frequently this way, without experiencing negative effects. Plain intermittent fasting—skipping breakfast altogether and fasting for a large portion of the day—can also work great, but it is more biologically stressful and harder to manage, especially if you have a demand-ing career and family. Bulletproof Intermittent Fasting helps manage these stresses for men and women alike, but based on anecdotal data, it is especially useful in addressing the interaction between fasting and sex hormones in women.

Instead of sending a stress signal reverberating through your body that you're starving, Bulletproof Intermittent Fasting basically tells your body to stay calm and designate resources for autophagy (cel-lular cleanup) and rapid fat burning (ketosis), but that it's not a fam-ine, either. You aren't taking in any starches or sugars, and there's no "famine stress" signal, so this style of intermittent fasting is unlikely to bring on adrenal fatigue. Your body uses the hormone epineph-rine (adrenaline) to burn fat, and epinephrine is made in your adrenal gland; reducing strain on the gland is especially important for women due to their sensitivity to adrenal burnout.

So what do you do on the days when you're not intermittent fasting? Have protein and fat in the morning, but not carbohydrates. Make a Bulletproof Coffee, and add some grass-fed collagen protein, 20 or 30 grams. Now breakfast is taken care of. It is not a fasting day because you had protein, so you are good to go do HIIT or lift weights (or just have a normal day!). Some women do well by eating normally all week and once a week doing a full twenty-four-hour fast. Take advantage of scheduling flexibility. Pick a low-stress day, skip breakfast, skip lunch, eat dinner. There, you did it!

In addition to lacing your fast with some MCT oil, I also recom-mend that you experiment with less aggressive fasting schedules. You might fast for fourteen or twelve hours instead of the full sixteen, for instance, or space your fasting days farther apart. If those fasts prove comfortable, you always have the option of adding hours and frequency. The key thing is to keep your hormones from going into panic mode. There is a reason that stressed women crave fatty and salty foods: they are experiencing a symptom of adrenal exhaustion. It's important to pay attention to these potentially serious symptoms and not treat them as another problem to overcome through sheer willpower. Part of exerting self-control through fasting is learning to distinguish superficial cravings from genuine warning signs.

The adrenals produce aldosterone, the hormone that balances sodium and potassium levels in the bloodstream. That balance is critical for proper cell function, so if you're feeling stressed, eating a little extra salt can help ease the burden on your overtaxed adrenals. Your body craves salty foods for a reason—listen to it! Add some mineral-rich Himalayan sea salt to your diet. (Pro tip: stir a pinch of Himalayan salt into a glass of water and drink it first thing in the morning.) This is an easy way to boost energy and help reduce adrenal stress, and your body needs more salt (2 to 8 grams a day) when you are in ketosis anyway. If you crave fat, add some fat to your diet. Just skip the potato chips and make it the good kind, like the fat in grass-fed butter, avocado, and olive oil.

Later in the day, if your body is still telling you that you need more salty foods, there's nothing like vegetables soaked in butter and sprinkled with high-quality sea salt. Or grass-fed steak prepared the same way! Flexible fasting isn't just a good idea, it's absolutely vital for your health. It helps you tap into the advantages of *going without* while protecting your adrenals and your fertility.

If you're a woman over forty and/or have significant weight to lose, here's a hack for you: before you start intermittent fasting, change your breakfast routine for about a month. Soon after you wake up, eat a morning meal with some fat (including MCT oil) and at least 40 grams of protein. It will reset your leptin sensitivity, making it easier to lose weight. You can have tea and a few eggs, a piece of meat, salmon and avocado, or whatever protein smoothie you like, as long as there are no carbs. After thirty days, do the every-other-day intermittent fasting schedule described above.

Women's bodies are more highly attuned to stress signals (again, for fertility reasons), which is why they benefit from their morning fat and often protein. Women also are more carbohydrate sensitive than men, on average. For this reason, I suggest establishing times between fasts when you replenish your body with carbs by eating more of them than you might normally. Many men thrive on having such a "carbohydrate refeed" day only once a week. Some men perform at their peak when they eat carbs even less frequently. Most women do exceptionally well eating low to medium amounts of carbs *at every dinner* instead of trying to stay in ketosis all the time. This carb-laced diet works because intermittent fasting, and the power of MCT to turn on mild ketones, is enough to get the benefits; meanwhile, the carbs are great for sleep and for sending a signal to your body that it can relax—there is no impending famine.

To be clear: when I'm talking about allowing some carbs, I'm not suggesting you go crazy with the bread and pizza. Stick to high-quality carbs such as sweet potatoes, carrots, squash, and white rice. *Do not* eat gluten, corn syrup, and processed carbs. They may cause inflammatory responses and will very likely make you feel tired the next day. They will definitely make you feel a bit heavier the next day, because your body will store extra glycogen, along with the water that comes with it. Don't worry, it's just water weight! You can't put on a pound of fat in one day no matter what you do. But even if you occasionally indulge in low-quality foods, it's not the end of the world. Eating junk food on refuel day will cause several days of cravings and lower performance, but you can bounce back. It's a long journey.

If you eat moderate amounts of red meat and organ meat, you're probably getting enough iron in your diet. Women generally need more iron than men, partly due to blood loss during menstruation. Some women need supplementary iron. Low blood levels of ferritin (an iron-transporting protein) disrupt the menstrual cycle, lead to fatigue, and contribute to an overall feeling of poor health. Many women of childbearing age are anemic because they don't get enough red meat in their diets, and this can cause complications during pregnancy.

Women need to pay special attention to iron. Too little is bad; too much can also cause trouble. Unlike vitamin D or K_2, iron isn't one of the supplements that you want to take randomly, no matter what. It's terrible for your performance to be anemic (low in iron), but taking enough iron to raise your blood ferritin level above about 75 micrograms per liter will age you really quickly. The best bet is to get your iron level tested to see if you need an iron supplement. You will have to ask your doctor to test specifically for ferritin, as most normal blood panels don't run this test. A lot of standard medical testing is still not tailored to women's physiology, unfortunately.

A woman's body begins seeking resources for the fetus practically from the moment of fertilization. I remember an incident from many years ago, when my wife and I were trying to start a family. The first time I was sure she was pregnant was when we ordered the last bowl of an amazing lamb stew at a restaurant in Lake Tahoe. There was one big piece of lamb in it, and we were sharing the bowl. I went to scoop it up, but she took her spoon and pushed mine out of the way. As I watched her savor every bite, I thought, "Oh, my God, she's pregnant!"

No matter what, if you eat too few calories over time, your body will get stressed in response to the famine signal and you may start having fertility problems until quality food supplies or caloric intake return to levels that support reproduction. That's an issue whether or not you are actually trying to start a family, because fertility is a proxy for good health status overall.

The starvation-stress response is one reason why women who are suffering from eating disorders often stop menstruating. Their bodies are in panic mode and are attempting to protect them from the additional stress of pregnancy by cutting off fertility. Controlled animal studies have documented just how extreme the response can be: when female rats were given an extremely low-calorie diet, they stopped their reproductive cycle and also developed a significantly heightened response to stress.[5] This is just one more reason why CICO diets built around calorie restriction are not a generally healthy practice.

I do not advocate intense daily exercise for men or women who are fasting unless they're pro athletes practicing intense recovery, too. Many female athletes—including "weekend warriors"—stop menstruating and are no longer fertile. It's very stressful to the body to combine extreme amounts of exercise with a low-fat, low-calorie diet. This sends a signal to your cellular epigenome that says, "You run all the time, so a tiger must be chasing you every single day. And there's obviously no food since you're not eating. Your life must be under threat by famine and tigers. Yikes! Don't get pregnant!!"

Both male and female bodies respond to these messages with exhaustion, adrenal fatigue, and hormone imbalances, but women are more sensitive to these problems and feel the effects first. A diet consisting of high healthy fats, moderate protein intake, and cyclical low carb intake is extremely healthy and beneficial. I have met many women (and men like me, too, of course) who have struggled with weight and "dieting" their entire adult lives, only to finally find a sustainable way of eating when they discovered intermittent fasting, cut out inflammatory foods, and started their morning with Bulletproof Coffee. Your personal carb threshold will vary, and only you have the power to figure it out using these guidelines.

Overall, if you're a woman, you need to exercise more caution than a man would in balancing your biology with the benefits of intermittent fasting. This is hugely important: NEVER FAST WHEN YOU ARE PREGNANT! I strongly suggest that you see a doctor before fasting if you fall into any of these categories:

- You are breastfeeding or planning to get pregnant.

- You have fertility problems or irregular periods.

- You are underweight or malnourished.

- You have a history of eating disorders.

Remember, fasting is a process, not a single act. Respect the process, approach it with care and dedication, and you will soon find yourself in a much better place.

THE OLDER GENERATION

There's a whole other aspect of fasting for women that I haven't talked about yet: the way it plays out for women who are past menopause. There are about 50 million women in the United States who fall into this category,[6] but you sure wouldn't know it by looking at the articles and studies about fasting. Older women are nearly invisible when it comes to fasting, which is not okay.

I have an up-close perspective on this topic, because my wife is at the end of perimenopause and she practices intermittent fasting with me. What we see—personally, anecdotally, and in the limited scientific literature—is that there's a tremendous range in the way women's bodies respond at and after menopause. I think the most important thing to point out is that everything shifts when you enter menopause, so inevitably your response to fasting is going to change as well. It may very well shift every month.

Everyone is susceptible to becoming addicted to fasting (what I call the "fasting trap"—more on that shortly), but women seem to be especially vulnerable, perhaps because there is so much social pressure to be thin. Compulsive fasting, like any other kind of addictive or craving-driven behavior, is not good for you. I hear stories from women all the time: The fasting made me feel really good. Then my sleep quality went away. Then my hair started to fall out. Then my menstrual cycle went bonkers. Often women don't recognize these as symptoms of the fasting trap, because the effects can resemble those of perimenopause.

When you reach perimenopause, your hair really is likely to get thinner, and some of it may fall out. You may experience hot flashes, anxiety, and changes in your sleeping behavior. Those changes may distract you from the ways you could be overdoing fasting. But even if you had developed a smart, balanced, flexible dieting plan for yourself before perimenopause, you are going to need to make some adjustments. Your body has a lot of new things going on. You want to be kind to yourself: face down your anxiety, yes, but through transcendence, not through suffering.

After menopause, after you've stabilized, you will probably do very well on intermittent fasting, possibly even better than before. My mother loves it, for instance. She does intermittent fasting and one meal a day (OMAD) almost all the time. It took her a while to get used to it, but now she says she feels much better when she fasts. For my wife, who is still in perimenopause, the effects of OMAD are more erratic. Some days she feels amazing, others not. The way you feel on any given day during a fast is also very much tied to where you are in your menstrual cycle, if you still have a cycle.

For women who are in menopause, you need to make a whole new self-assessment. Take a good look at how metabolically fit you currently are. If you are average, the answer is probably "not very fit at all." You can actually start out gently by just skipping breakfast and having a Bulletproof Coffee. No proteins or carbs for breakfast—a little bit of *going without*. Maybe the first day you will have a whole stick of grass-fed butter with your coffee. Just live it up. Does that sound odd? Once you try it, you'll be a believer. It's like a hot milk-shake. If that feels like too much fat at the beginning of the day, you can back off.

Tell yourself, "I'm just going to go until lunch." Okay. All you did was skip breakfast. You can do this. Then you increase the size of your fasting window. You get it up to a sixteen-hour fast. Now you have dinner maybe around 6:00 p.m. Then you go without eating till 6:00 a.m. That's twelve hours. Now go another six. That's lunchtime. You'll be okay. Moving around also helps a lot. It's very doable.

Once you've got that solid foundation, start eating gently. Once you've got that going, you want to move into a longer rhythm, like an ongoing 16:8 fast. The basic rules of fasting are the same for everyone, men and women, premenopausal and postmenopausal. It's really in the fine-tuning that women in perimenopause and beyond need to make special allowances. Things that worked for you a few years ago might not work so well anymore. If you're feeling worse than you did before, the fast might not be the cause—but it might. Adjusting the way you fast might also be part of your solution to boosting your energy and focus and reducing your stress and anxiety.

In general, if you are entering perimenopause, try shorter intermittent fasts, and don't do them back to back until you are sure they are working for you. This is to minimize the chances of accidentally making any symptoms you have worse! Drinking alcohol, even a glass of wine, may make fasting harder. I recommend seeing a doctor and getting a hormone and thyroid panel done to assess your health and get a clearer picture of what you are working with. Changes in body composition and weight are a normal part of menopause and are not just the results of your diet. Even if you do the world's most perfect intermittent fasting plan and eat all the best-quality foods, an under-functioning thyroid will still make you put on weight. The changes in your estrogen-to-progesterone ratio can also make weight loss challenging.

I don't need to tell you that it's okay and normal for the appearance of your body to change as it ages; there is nothing to apologize for there. But even if weight loss isn't your goal or losing weight has become challenging, I still recommend intermittent fasting. It will help you maintain muscle tone and fight the loss of bone density that can lead to osteoporosis. Recent research has also revealed that intermittent fasting helps increase a molecule called kisspeptin and stimulates your ovaries and adrenals to make estrogen and progesterone[7]—which can help ease the symptoms of menopause.

The bottom line here is that women are not just men with wombs, even though a lot of the popular writing about diet and fasting might make you think they are. Women define our challenges and potentials as a species every bit as much as men do. When you plan your diet, sleep, exercise, supplements, and all of the other things that go into your fast, be mindful of the cycles and the sex-specific evolutionary legacy you carry inside you. Don't deprive yourself of resources if you are planning to get pregnant. Never fast during pregnancy. Talk to your doctor as your body enters the changes of menopause.

But be mindful, too, of the creative and procreative sides of your evolutionary legacy. They are part of the strength you can draw upon as you experiment with ways to *go without*, take control, and release your better self.

10

FAST *EVERY* WAY:
A HOW-TO GUIDE

For four days, I had struggled through hunger, loneliness, fear, and anxiety. Then, on the final morning of the vision quest, I woke to a glorious sound: peaceful silence. The bees were still doing buzzy loops around my head. The little brown bird was still thrashing about in the pile of brush I'd arranged at the entrance to the cave. No, the silence I was hearing was coming from inside of me: I couldn't hear the voice in my head. "There's no food. You're going to starve," it had lied to me. "You're alone, so you're going to die." Finally it had shut up.

I had been on enough journeys like this that I knew that each experience is different and spiritual progress is an unpredictable thing. It's far more likely to sneak up on you than to come at you directly. You can capture it as long as you're ready and willing to let it in whenever and wherever it happens to show up. In this case, my mental state had begun to shift only after I managed to appreciate the absurdity of the things that had so tormented me over the past couple days. The bees weren't actually harming me. The bird was not a mountain lion ready to attack. I realized that there had been a lot of silliness going on in my head. I had believed my own stories.

Beneath the silliness were the more serious cravings and the yearnings that had driven me to go on this vision quest in the first place. So much of what I was feeling was rooted in my relationship to food. Food is tied up with fear, and it's tied up with loneliness, and it's tied up with culture and family and what you did with your parents growing up and even how your mother fed you as a baby. These kinds of things live inside all of us, incubating and growing from the moment we're born, and they're not born from the world of thoughts. They tend to lurk far below the conscious level, but they sure do manage to make their presence known. To become the kind of person I had chosen to be, I had decided to deal with all of that.

I meditated for hours inside my cave. Eventually I got tired of waiting for a vision. Or had I already had one? I got up and hiked around a few of the amazing canyons that carve their way through the Sonoran Desert. I stacked up rocks into cairns, poked a cactus, and meditated some more. The vision quest was nearly over. Pretty soon Delilah would come rolling along in her battered old pickup to take me home.

I'd done it. I'd made it four days alone, without food, and I didn't feel terrible or tired. Actually, I felt more in control than I had in a long time, maybe ever. I felt bulletproof, even though I had not yet birthed my company by that name. For the first time, I understood that the greatest gift of fasting is that it helps you divorce your story about food from the reality of your biology. My journey had given me four days of open time to examine and unpack my stupid belief systems about food. So many of the things I had blindly accepted as the way of the world were merely the result of cultural and dietary training. Social events don't have to be built around eating and drinking (but it's okay if they are). You don't have to eat three meals a day. You can be in control of your hunger, rather than the other way around.

It was shocking to look in the mirror after I returned from my vision quest. My face looked different. My pants were way looser. I stepped on the scale and was baffled to see that the needle was 20 pounds lighter than before. That couldn't be right. I knew I wasn't dehydrated. After drinking normal amounts of water for the four days, I wasn't thirsty at all, despite the dry desert air. I had so much water left over that I poured some out of my canteen when I left the cave.

And there was no way I could have shed 20 pounds of fat in four days. Biologically—unless you've had liposuction—you can't do that. I had lost, maybe, a couple pounds of fat. So where was the rest of me?

What really happened, I now know, was that my body lost a whole lot of inflammation *and* I had turned on ketosis. When you go into ketosis, you can easily lose 10 pounds during the first week by shedding stored glycogen along with all the water it was bound to. At the same time, I had stopped eating all food, including the foods that cause inflammation in my tissues, and started filling my body with anti-inflammatory ketones. When that inflammation went away, I dropped a lot more water weight. My whole metabolism changed in response. The vision quest was one of the first times in my life that I felt the incredible burst of energy that comes with fasting. I also felt an elevated state of mental clarity and physical lack of soreness in the joints of my back and knees, even the knee that's had three surgeries. My body had switched into "go mode," and I wanted to feel that way all the time.

YOUR CYCLES OF LIFE

For me, the end of the vision quest was the beginning of my new relationship with food and, by extension, my new relationship with myself. For you, the end of reading about fasting is the beginning of actually doing it. There is a beautiful circularity to fasting, as there is with life in general. We breathe in and out in cycles. We eat and drink in cycles of metabolism as well. According to one famous estimate from Oak Ridge National Laboratory, 98 percent of the atoms in your body are replaced every year.[1] Almost all of your cells are replaced every seven years. Matter moves through you, energy moves through you, yet somehow you remain *you*—ideally, a steadily improving version of you, but you all the same.

The circularity of it all reminds me of the ouroboros, one of the oldest symbols in mythology. You've probably seen one—it is a snake coiled around to form a circle, eating its own tail. The ouroboros made its first known appearance on the sarcophagus of King Tutankhamen in Egypt more than three thousand years ago. To the Egyptians, the ouroboros represented an endless process of renewal. Plato later wrote about it and said the same thing. To the early Christian mystics, it evoked the merging of the physical and spiritual worlds. And to the medieval alchemists, the ouroboros was emblematic of the search for spiritual transcendence.

An essential part of the fasting process is finding the specific version of the cycle that works for you. Every person has a different state of health, different goals, different cravings to overcome. The biggest takeaway here is that *there is no one-size-fits-all approach to fasting*. To get the most out of fasting, you'll need to know the wide range of techniques and hacks you can draw from. Take time to find the perfect fit, pay attention to how you feel, and don't be afraid to experiment with different schedules. Be willing to fail at a fast. Be willing to suffer. Be willing to choose *not* to suffer. Think of this as part of your journey of self-discovery. It's an expression of your uniqueness: not just your biological state but also all of the pains and pleasures and aspirations that belong to you alone.

By now you know that if you don't eat anything for more than fourteen hours, you're fasting. Longer fasts work better. You can fast to lose weight and fix your metabolism. You can fast to heal your gut. You can fast for personal growth and spiritual states. Heck, you can even have a few types of calories while fasting and get the same results. You are ready to start exploring and gaining control. Still, there are some common types of fasts that are either particularly easy to fit into your schedule or have been promoted enough that they have about the same meaning when you talk with others about fasting. Here is the complete list.

THE 16:8 FAST

This is the foundational style of intermittent fasting. The name refers to the pattern of eating and fasting hours: you consume all of your daily calories within a shortened period (typically around eight hours) and fast the rest of the time (sixteen hours). Some people call it the

"Leangains Method," which is not accurate. (Leangains is a program[2] developed by Martin Berkhan for strength athletes that uses a 16:8 fast, along with other techniques.) The simplest way to do a 16:8 fast is to reduce your pattern to two meals a day. Women may want to do a slightly shortened version; see below. A typical routine might look like this:

1. Skip breakfast and start your day without food. You may instinctively already do this.

2. Around noon, break your fast and have your first meal.

3. Eat dinner based on whatever eating style you like—it doesn't have to be keto.

4. Stop eating by 8:00 p.m. to allow plenty of time for digestion before you go to sleep.

5. Repeat this schedule the next day.

If you're a purist, you might drink nothing but water during your fast, but you can also have black coffee or tea.

BULLETPROOF INTERMITTENT FASTING

This one is my go-to fast, and it will probably be yours as well for the reasons described in previous chapters. It uses a fast of at least 16:8 (or longer), but with one crucial biohack to make your fast easier and more effective: *drink a cup of Bulletproof Coffee in the morning.* The medium-chain triglycerides (MCT) and high-quality fats from grass-fed butter keep you feeling full until lunch, yet they also allow your body to continue autophagy and fat-burning so you get all the benefits of intermittent fasting. You can add a tiny dollop of butter and a dash of C8 MCT oil, or you can go bigger if you have a big day. Yes, you're really fasting!

I came up with Bulletproof Intermittent Fasting ten years ago to address the one huge downside of regular intermittent fasting: it can leave you feeling hungry, tired, and distracted, especially when you're first getting started. It's hard to focus on crushing your to-do list when your brain is constantly thinking about lunch. To get the benefits of intermittent fasting, you need to stick with it and power through the initial feelings of fatigue. All too often, those hunger pangs cause people to give up, because we have jobs to do, kids to raise, errands to run, or other responsibilities to attend to while we're fasting.

Bulletproof Intermittent Fasting solves a lot of those problems and helps ease newbies into the world of fasting. When you start your morning with a cup of Bulletproof Coffee, the fats push your body into a mild state of ketosis, which curbs your cravings and fuels you with energy-rich ketones all morning long. Best of all, it does these things without switching on protein or sugar digestion and all of the chemical work that goes with it. By avoiding carbs and proteins, you continue to reap the benefits of a fasted state—without feeling like a hungry zombie.

If you want to make sure that you've optimized your Bulletproof fast, you can easily test your ketone levels at home. Ketone testing strips are sold online, as well as in most pharmacies. They're simple to use: they change color according to the number of ketones in your urine, which tells you if you're slightly in ketosis or deep in ketosis. The magic ketone number you want to hit is 0.48 mmol/L, but the affordable "pee strips" won't give exact numbers. For that, you will need to buy a far more accurate Precision Xtra ketone meter. You prick your finger as you would for a blood sugar test, get a pinhead-sized drop of blood, and stick a test strip into the meter. It provides a very precise digital measurement of your blood ketone levels. It will make sense as soon as you get your hands on a kit.

First test your ketone levels to get a baseline. Then make your Bulletproof Coffee, starting with one teaspoon of Brain Octane MCT oil in your coffee (Brain Octane MCT oil raises ketones more than normal MCT oil does), drink it, then test your ketone levels forty-five minutes later to see the spike. Gradually increase the Brain Octane MCT oil you take over the next few weeks until your ketone level is above 0.48 mmol/L. Then see how you feel: Are you able to power through your morning without thinking about lunch? If not, you can keep adjusting.

A typical day of Bulletproof Intermittent Fasting might go like this:

1. Drink a cup of Bulletproof Coffee in the morning instead of eating breakfast. No sugar, no cream, no fake creamer, no artificial sweetener.

2. Either skip lunch for a longer intermittent fast, or eat a late lunch according to your food template (bonus points and faster progress come from using the Bulletproof Fasting Roadmap at daveasprey.com/fasting).

3. Finish eating by 7:00 to 8:00 p.m.

4. Repeat this schedule every day or just a few times per week. Remember, your body hates strict routine, so feel free to mix it up.

THE 5:2 FAST

In this case, the numbers refer to days rather than hours. On a 5:2 fast, you eat normally five days a week. On the other two days, you drastically reduce your intake to between 500 and 600 calories. This sort of fast is focused primarily on weight loss, which is why it is sometimes called the "Fast Diet."

There is good evidence that people lose weight on this diet. However, given that you can eat whatever you want on the days when you're "fasting," you're unlikely to get the benefits of autophagy. The only thing you're really *going without* is lots of calories on two days of the week.

There are no standard guidelines for what to eat on your fasting/dieting days. Obviously, you want to go for the highest-quality foods that fit into your diet (not 600 calories of potato chips!), but some form of fasting is always better than no fasting at all. You can also experiment with when you want to take your calories on fasting days, as long as you don't do it close to bedtime. You might want to take three very small meals, though you will probably have better results by bundling your calories into just lunch and dinner.

The 5:2 fast is broadly similar to alternate-day fasting, which is exactly what it sounds like. Because alternate-day fasting is straightforward to test in the lab, it's used in many studies of the effects of intermittent fasting. Some of the well-documented health benefits[3] include weight loss, reduced insulin resistance, reduced allergies,[4] decreased inflammation, decreased oxidative stress,[5] better cardiovascular health,[6] and overall improved metabolic fitness. Note that these benefits are not unique to alternate-day fasting. You will achieve them in most if not all forms of intermittent fasting.

ONE MEAL A DAY (OMAD)

In this fasting plan, you eat one meal a day. Calling it OMAD sounds more badass, though, so that's what most people do. Strangely, when you tell someone you are eating only one meal a day, they don't react nearly as strongly as if you say you're fasting. It's because they hear that you are eating, instead of going without. In OMAD, you consume all of your daily calories in a single meal and fast the rest of the day.

In other words, OMAD is a 23:1 fast, which gives your body twenty-three hours each day to reap the benefits of a fasting lifestyle. If you're looking to burn fat, improve mental resilience, and minimize the amount of time you spend on your food schedule (you know, if meal prep and eating feel bothersome to you), you should investigate this one. Of course, if you did 22:2, or 20:4, you would also get the same basic benefits. So it's a bit silly to single out the twenty-four-hour OMAD fast with a special name, but if sounding badass helps get you into fasting mode—embrace it.

For most people, between 4:00 and 7:00 p.m. is an ideal time to break the fast with your daily meal. That window gives you fuel when you need it most; it also provides a time to eat socially with friends or family and leaves enough time to digest your food before heading to bed. Intermittent fasting schedules above 16:8, such as OMAD, activate stress response pathways that boost mitochondrial performance, autophagy, and the repair of the DNA in your cells, as well as reducing the risk of chronic disease.[7] The extra few hours beyond 16:8 do provide additional benefits.

On the other hand, OMAD can be a pretty extreme intermittent fasting schedule if you do it every day, especially if you are new to fasting. Avoiding food for twenty-three hours a day takes a lot of effort, and if it stresses you out, you will lose some of the powerful benefits of fasting. It's also especially challenging for women for all of the hormonal reasons discussed in chapter 9. The goal here isn't to feel as though you're punishing your body or suffering through a challenge. Fasting does not need to include suffering—unless you want it to. A successful transition to intermittent fasting requires training your body to handle a new routine and then working to make it sustainable. In general, I recommend doing OMAD no more than three times a week.

I often find that when I do a 16:8 Bulletproof Intermittent Fast, when lunchtime rolls around, I'm not hungry. So I skip it. By dinnertime, I've magically completed a 23:1 OMAD fast. It's much harder to wake up and tell yourself, "Today I'm doing an OMAD fast," than it is to tell yourself at lunch, "Hey, if I just wait six more hours for dinner, I am in OMAD land!"

Here are a few tips to get the most out of an OMAD fasting plan:

1. Introduce intermittent fasting every other day.

2. Start by fasting in shorter durations. Get comfortable fasting for sixteen to twenty hours at a time, and slowly build up to fasting for twenty-three hours a day.

3. Try one 23:1 day, then add more, at most three, OMAD days into your weekly routine. As with any style of fasting, it's important to see how your body responds and find what works for you.

4. Eat according to your food template; OMAD works with all of them, but most people on OMAD choose to limit the amount of carbs in their diets or to eat according to the Bulletproof Fasting Roadmap at daveasprey.com/fasting. When you eat a lot of carbohydrates, your body stockpiles glucose as glycogen and it takes a lot longer for your body to shift into ketosis. You can also modify OMAD to include a cup of Bulletproof Coffee in the morning, which is a great hack to have more energy during the day, or with prebiotic fiber, which is a hack to keep you from being hungry while feeding good gut bacteria.

5. Make your one meal count: balanced and diverse, with a full range of macro- and micronutrients.

6. Adjust the schedule. If it's more comfortable for you to spread your large meal out over more than an hour, do it. Maintaining your composure (and your sanity) is more important than a strict timeline.

7. Break your fast mindfully. After fasting all day, you may feel that you want to eat the biggest meal possible as quickly as possible—not a good idea because you'll feel sick at first. That said, the goal of intermittent fasting is not to limit your calorie intake. If you normally consume 2,000 calories in a day, you can eat a 2,000-calorie dinner of high-quality, high-calorie food.

8. Listen to your body, and recognize when to stop. OMAD may simply not agree with your metabolism, your exercise regimen, or your lifestyle. That's okay. Don't force a schedule without listening to your body's cues. If you're not sleeping well, or if you're feeling sluggish, weak, or constantly tired, your body is telling you that it needs more energy more often.

9. Women should be especially attentive to their responses to an OMAD diet. Studies show that excessive intermittent fasting can interfere with women's insulin response.[8] If you notice

negative changes in how you feel or shifts in your menstrual cycle, fast less. See a doctor for a hormone test if things don't level out as they should.

Remember that fasting can cause more than just physical stress. *This is true of all types of fasting*, but especially of OMAD because it is the longest fast you can do in one day. Restricting yourself to one meal a day can be taxing to your mind if you obsess over food all day. Take care of your stress levels by practicing yoga, meditating, exercising—really, whatever helps you find your Zen. You are not in a race. You are not trying to prove something. More difficult fasts do not equal better results; they won't automatically get you there more quickly. Make sure that your schedule feels right, and keep in mind that it's fine to try different styles of fasting and to take breaks from fasting entirely.

OTHER TYPES OF FASTING

People have recently become very creative in inventing and naming new styles of fasting. That's a good thing—it means that lots of folks are experimenting and personalizing their strategies—but all the terms can get a little confusing, especially when you start googling fasting. So in the hope of dispelling some of that confusion, let's look at some of the other most popular fasting methods. I recommend starting with the 16:8 intermittent fast and then working up from there.

Spontaneous meal skipping: Strictly speaking, this is not fasting, but it is a great way to prepare your mind and body for a more regimented approach to fasting. Simply skip a meal now and then, overriding the hunger pains and that silly voice telling you that you're going to starve to death. If you live a hectic lifestyle, you may do this sometimes already. When you skip meals deliberately, you begin to break the habit of eating because it's "mealtime." Then you allow your body to learn to *go without* from time to time, just as our ancestors did for many thousands of years. This style of fasting will not put you into ketosis, and it won't turn on autophagy, but it *will* increase your cortisol level as your body uses it to generate some blood sugar quickly. When your metabolism is flexible and working well, this won't be an issue for you.

Crescendo fast: This is the gentlest form of intermittent fasting. It is basically a 16:8 fast, but you fast only every other day, and on fasting days you don't exercise strongly.

Eat stop eat: The primary focus of this fast is two twenty-four-hour periods of complete fasting per week, generally lasting from one dinner to the next. Then you would eat normally the other five days of the week, alternating days so that you never have two fast days in a row. You may be asking yourself what the difference is between eat stop eat and just doing OMAD twice per week. The answer is . . . good marketing! They're the same thing. Eat stop eat is different from 5:2 fasting because on fasting days, you actually fast with eat stop eat, and on 5:2 you're allowed to consume 600 calories. Many people, including me, start OMAD with a cup of Bulletproof Coffee.

Alternate-day fast: As the name suggests, this program has you fasting for twenty-four hours every other day. Some people prefer to go completely without food on fast days, while others eat minimally, restricting their intake to a few hundred calories, in the style of the 5:2 fast. This is another pretty extreme approach that is not recommended for fasting newcomers. I would also not recommend doing alternate-day fasting for extended periods of time because it places too much stress on the body.

Now we come to a couple truly extreme versions of fasting.

Water fast: Should you drink nothing but water during a fast? I would recommend against this unless it's part of a spiritual journey for you. Most water fasts are one to three days long and allow no other liquid or food. People tend to combat their hunger pangs by overdoing it on the water, chugging multiple liters a day. You simply must add salt or electrolytes to the water, or you can get sick or even die. Some people do up to ten-day water fasts, but you should attempt that only under medical supervision. Since you are eliminating calories entirely, you will lose a lot of weight, but you may also suffer from dizziness and a significant drop in blood pressure, technically known as orthostatic hypotension. Strangely, a water fast may also leave you dehydrated, because a lack of bulk in your colon means your colon can't absorb liquid the way it normally does.

Extended fast: It is generally considered safe to go up to four or five days of fasting without needing any sort of special accommodations. Some people will do up to ten days, but a four-day fast, like the one I did in the cave, is more common. During an extended fast, you would not eat any sugar, artificial sweetener, or any other form of carbohydrate or starch or any form of protein. Even healthy protein will definitely break the fast. The longer the fast, the more important it is to maintain your electrolytes, the critical electrically charged minerals in your body. An electrolyte drink shouldn't be a sugary sports drink. What you really want is to get your essential doses of magnesium, calcium, sodium, and small amounts of potassium. A zero-calorie electrolyte drink mix is your best bet. At a very minimum, put a pinch of salt into your water. When I do an extended fast for up to five days, I usually have Bulletproof Coffee on the first two or three days and switch to black coffee in the morning after my body is fully adapted to the fast.

At the other end of the spectrum are quasi-fasting diets that have health and psychological benefits, even though they don't involve a full break from digestion. These include the following.

Protein fasting: I introduced this concept ten years ago in *The Bulletproof Diet*. Once a week, you consume no more than 15 grams of protein in an entire twenty-four-hour period. Studies show that restricting your protein intake to near zero will turn on autophagy. This is hard to do, because even most vegetables have some protein in them, and those little bits add up quickly. You end up eating some rice, some coconut milk, and some veggies for a day, usually about 1,000 calories. This approach is fantastic if you want to eat on a social occasion, because you can easily transform an intermittent fasting 16:8 day into a protein-fasting day by having a light lunch and dinner. Or you could just do an OMAD fast, which definitely contains less than 15 grams of protein. In practice, OMAD is easier to do because it requires less thinking than a protein fast does. On the other hand, a protein fast lets you feel less deprived and be more social. One day a week is fine, and it stacks well with anything from 16:8 to OMAD.

Fasting-mimicking diet: This eating plan tricks your body into thinking it is fasting, even though you eat specific low-carb, low-protein, high-fat foods for five consecutive days. Some people like to criticize this approach and say that it's not really a fast. Here's my take: if it does the same thing, or most of the same things, as a fast, it's a fast but probably not a gut-healing fast. A recent study by gerontologist Min Wei and his colleagues at the University of Southern California found that the fasting-mimicking diet is highly effective for weight loss.[9] It is likely to be less effective at activating autophagy than the other fasting techniques discussed here. But for all the other reasons you would fast, including longevity, fasting mimicking is legit. The only reason people say it's not a fast is because of a misguided, puritanical belief that fasting should make you miserable.

The fasting-mimicking diet allows up to 400 calories a day several days in a row, which is why you get a lot of the benefits of fasting. You're consuming fewer calories than normal during that time, and I would argue more satiety, the feeling of being full. Don't fall into the trap that says fasting has to be 0 calories or else it's not a fast. That is not how fasting actually works. If you're getting the results of fasting, including weight loss and metabolic benefits, and feel stronger and more in control, that's cool. Suffering, on the other hand? Not cool.

Seasonal eating: This is a pleasantly primal method of eating, focused on eating only foods that are available each season. Summer is a time of eating fresh fruit and vegetables, with more carbs and little if any fasting, while winter has more fasting and is mostly keto, based on the idea that our ancestors could hunt in winter but had little ability to store lots of carbs for winter. You can combine seasonal eating with any of the patterns of fasting. Mainly, this approach is a good way to steer yourself toward eating fresh, unprocessed foods—which generally happen to be both delicious and healthy.

Dopamine fast: This falls into the broad category of nonfood fasts that I mentioned earlier. The purpose of a dopamine fast is to abstain from anything that causes your body to secrete dopamine, a neurotransmitter that is closely associated with our pleasure sensors and can play a role in reinforcing addictions. Eating spicy or sweet food causes a dopamine spike. So does having lots of social interaction, in person or on social media. Just about all of life's pleasures give you a dopamine hit: gaming, watching TV or pornography, gambling, shopping, and having sex. Oh, and drugs and alcohol. The intent of a dopamine fast isn't to make yourself miserable, it's to allow your dopamine receptors to take a break so that when they come back online, they'll become more sensitive to dopamine. When you stop the fast, which normally lasts two to seven days, you will find that everything you do feels more pleasurable. Training your body to *go without* all of its various cravings will make you stronger and more directed. My fasting in a cave for four days was an intense dopamine fast, among other things.

THE FASTING TRAP

I've just spent almost an entire book sharing everything I know about fasting and extolling its virtues. Now take a minute to balance out that elation with a cautionary note about what I call the "fasting trap." It's a consequence of the natural habit formation pathways in our brains. Pay attention, because to get the most out of fasting you need to beware of this trap.

Once upon a time, I was a raw vegan. That meant not eating any food or products coming from animals, no processed foods, and no foods cooked at temperatures above 118 degrees in the belief that foods are more nutritious if they are only minimally cooked—hence, the "raw" part. At first I felt amazing. After about six weeks, I lost some weight. I thought the diet was miraculous, so I committed to it completely.

It turned out that six weeks is a very significant number. B. J. Fogg at Stanford University, a behavioral scientist who specializes in studying habit formation, has shown that six weeks is the amount of time it takes to form a habit. (In the Bible, many significant events and fasts last forty days and forty nights, which is suspiciously similar to six weeks. People have had an intuitive feel for this process for a very long time.) Soon after that, my raw vegan habit started not working so well anymore. My body started to feel strange. My teeth became temperature sensitive, and then I cracked a tooth. I was cold all the time. I started getting new joint pain and new allergies. But I didn't stop, because I knew how good I felt on the diet.

To fix my problems, I decided, I needed to be an *even more committed* raw vegan. Obviously I wasn't committed enough! But things only got worse. I became really unhealthy, damaged my thyroid, and my joints started creaking. My memory became impaired. Eventually, I realized that lifestyle just wasn't working for me anymore. I had to undo the damage done to my body.

After that, I was determined to develop my own healthier and more constructive way to eat so I would never be fat again and never have the energy crashes that had plagued me my entire life, including all through the vegan time. That was the birth of my Bulletproof Diet. Along the way, I learned that going into ketosis can have some of the same habit-forming risks as a diet like raw vegan. In the late 1990s, when I was first experimenting with fasting, I tried the Atkins diet—or dirty keto, as it's called today. This protein-heavy, high-fat diet put the body into ketosis, which I loved. I ate a steak every night and really restricted my carb intake. I lost half the weight I wanted to, felt the glow of success, and became convinced that that was the only way to do it.

When my weight loss stalled, I resolved to be even more keto, not understanding that I was inflaming my body by eating the wrong foods. By that point, my ego was so bound up in succeeding that I didn't want to admit I needed to rethink my entire approach. I was also a victim of what behavioral scientists call the "sunk cost fallacy." I couldn't get my time and effort back, so I was determined to put in even more time and effort until I succeeded. It's the same psychological glitch that convinces people to keep investing more money into failing businesses or to continue gambling to make up for their ever-mounting losses. You may know the common saying "throwing good money after bad." It never leads to success, and it sure didn't work for me while I was doing the wrong kind of diet.

My troubles with the raw vegan and Atkins diets—aka the vegan trap and the keto trap—had a lot in common. If you do something for six weeks and it feels good, you tend to get hooked. At that point, you stop questioning whether it works. You keep doing it even if it messes with your health. People who eat dirty keto without breaks end up dropping their sex hormone levels, shedding hair, and ruining their sleep. People who go raw vegan get oxalic acid poisoning in their tissues and break the cell membranes in their brains by missing out on fatty acids from animals. They feel good and lose weight in the short term, so they get hooked on the habit. By the time allergies and metabolic dysfunction kick in, it's hard for them to stop.

Getting short-term benefits for six weeks makes you think that a strategy will always work—and just like me, you'll double down on something once you believe in it. It's a function of how people make decisions.

When I first started writing about intermittent fasting a decade ago, it was fairly esoteric knowledge. Some of the early Bulletproof followers, especially younger men, got very excited that they had found something new and powerful. They would say they were committing to doing intermittent fasting every day for the rest of their lives. Having been in two diet traps already, that made me nervous. So I'd like to pause for a moment and specifically address younger readers.

If you are eighteen to twenty-five years old, you probably have abundant energy (unless you have a serious illness or a metabolic dysfunction as I had at that age), so you can handle all kinds of self-destructive behaviors without feeling the consequences. You can go out drinking four nights a week, you can smoke or vape, and the next day you don't feel terrible. You can eat a bunch of junk food and brag, "I don't know how I do it, but I stay thin." None of those is a good idea, and you probably know that, but you can do them without having to reckon with the consequences right away.

In the same way, the resilience of youth may make intermittent fasting feel a little *too* easy. Strange as it sounds, you might enjoy it so much that you're tempted to do it frequently, which will create too much strain on your body over time. Creating an obsessive habit is never a good idea, even if it is an obsessive habit about intermittent fasting. You can overdo it, just as you can with any other type of behavior. Don't fall into the fasting trap.

The solution to the fasting trap is self-awareness. Expanding your self-awareness is one of the main goals of fasting anyway, so it's really important to work on it. If you do decide you're going to fast all the time, take a pause. STOP. Consciously consider that there is a serious risk of fasting too much. You don't want to fast when you're in physical pain, such as when you're sick or injured. The pain response chews through calories, making it hard to fast. If you're really addicted, you may be tempted to double down. STOP.

Every type of fast can do fantastic things for you. There's nothing wrong with going all in and doing one meal a day, which is a very powerful form of fasting. But here's the deal: even if you think of yourself as super-OMAD, every couple of weeks on Saturday, have some damn gluten-free waffles for breakfast.

If you're under eighteen, I urge special caution and restraint with fasting. Your body is still growing. Your brain's critical prefrontal cortex is not fully baked until about twenty-four years of age. An intermittent fast done one to three times a week, with adequate calories at the end of the fast, can provide benefits. But daily OMAD or daily 16:8 fasting can stunt your growth or your brain development. It's not worth the risk. You need high-quality food, and you need to send a strong signal to your body that there is zero risk of a famine. Long fasts may change your epigenetic signaling in a negative way that can take years to undo.

BREAK THE RULES *AND* BREAK THE FAST

Don't be afraid to break the fast. The nature of life is cycles—think of the ouroboros—and if you teach your body to exist in one constant state, whether it's a constant state of hunger or a constant state of carbohydrate access, you are training for weakness. You have to be able to eat flexibly, and you have to be able to handle your carbs.

People on long-term ketogenic diets and low-carb diets such as Atkins become insulin resistant over time, until they can't handle carbohydrates at all. That's not healthy or strong—in fact, it's as damaging to your body as eating sugar and carbs all the time! Generally, I don't eat breakfast—it's a pattern that works well for me. But I will tell you, after more than ten years of doing this, that sometimes on Saturdays I have a nice breakfast with my family, even one containing carbs, because it tastes good. My body can handle it, because it's become metabolically flexible.

I urge you not to become one of those inflexible people who thinks that you can turn away from carbs and never have to deal with them again. Don't be a fasting puritan or a fascist or whatever word you want to use for it. This is real life. It is full of curveballs and unexpected pleasures. You have to be ready for anything. And I'm here to make sure you are. Imagine if I were a purist and said, "I'm just going to have my Bulletproof Coffee for breakfast, and maybe if I'm really hungry, I'll put some collagen protein in there—but I'm never going to have waffles." You know what? That behavior would actually make me weaker. If you find yourself going down the path of perfection, it's time to spend a week on a "perfection fast" in which you deliberately eat imperfectly and go without fasting.

It's a discipline to have some kindness for yourself and to also allow yourself some rule bending. Strange as it seems, a lot of people don't believe in allowing simple pleasures into their lives. They equate rigor with achievement, and they never really live life as a result. The trap is that they get to the point where suffering feels good, so they keep doing it despite the costs. People who fast all the time will have exactly the same experience as people who are in keto all the time: a reduction in sex hormones, a reduction in thyroid hormone, an increase in cortisol and adrenaline, and a reduction in muscle mass.

Part of what makes the fasting trap so sinister is that nothing happens right away when you first fall in. Then, over time, the body pushes back. This is why it's vital that you find balance in your fasting lifestyle.

THE IMMUNITY FAST

Given the wave of concern over the past few years about new and resurgent infectious diseases, people often raise concerns about whether fasting is a good or a bad thing when you are sick. The COVID-19 pandemic really brought those questions to the surface. Here's the short answer: if you are metabolically flexible because you do regular fasting, your odds of getting extremely sick from any virus or bacterium decrease dramatically, because you are more resilient and have a healthier immune system. This is a powerful real-world example of what happens if you fast based on a balanced plan, strengthening your body and your mind without falling into the fasting trap.

Even if you have an active bacterial infection, studies show that avoiding carbohydrates and fasting enough to generate ketones is a good idea. You can recover more quickly if you don't eat carbohydrates, especially sugar—with one really important caveat. If you fast for a long period of time, your immune system may not have enough energy to mount the ideal response. (This is yet another example of why obsessive fasting is not a good idea.) In this case, moderate protein and energy from fats are going to be a good idea. On the other hand, if you have a viral infection, studies show that glucose in your bloodstream helps you recover faster. But to be clear: you don't have permission to pound a doughnut because you have the sniffles!

If you have a viral infection, eating moderate or even slightly higher amounts of protein, some slower-metabolizing starches, and maybe a few grams of glucose or sucrose could be good for you. Don't overdo it with the sugars, though. It is well established that drinking a lot of fruit juice or soda or eating high-sugar foods can dramatically lower your immune function. In any case, having ketones present in the body is anti-inflammatory and always a good idea. During a bacterial infection, you can achieve this state through diet alone. During a viral infection, a moderate carbohydrate intake is beneficial, so the only way to have ketones present when you eat carbs is to use MCT oil or have a Bulletproof Coffee in the morning.

Flexibility and adaptability are essential parts of being strong. That's true all the time, especially if you are already battling an infection. That's why you want to practice moderate amounts of fasting, so you will remain resilient.

To summarize: If you have a bacterial infection, avoid carbs and continue moderate fasting. If you have a viral infection, eat protein, eat a moderate amount of carbs but not sugar, and use MCT oil. And especially during high-stress times, don't give in to fear and despair. You have control over these things. You will be stronger and more resistant if you are in a good place psychologically as well as physically. Fasting can help with all of that.

Embrace life's variety. Don't fight the cycles of the world. And then you will sidestep the fasting trap and keep walking happily along your chosen path.

CONCLUSION: FAST IN PEACE

When I took my final hike around First Woman cave, my brain was on fire. Despite the desert heat and the rough terrain, I felt supercharged, as though I had a source of energy inside my body that hardly seemed possible. In hindsight, going off on my own along difficult, unfamiliar trails was a really bad idea. Terrible things could have happened if I'd gotten lost without enough water. But I was so charged that I had to move. Having that much energy violated my scientific understanding of the relationship between calories and metabolism. How could I be so powered up if I hadn't eaten anything? Clearly there was lot more going on in my body—emotionally, psychologically, and biologically—than I had been taught.

In my elevated state, I felt so good that I decided I didn't need my shaman to come get me. I texted Delilah, "Don't worry, I'll just walk back to the other cave. You can pick me up there. I have way too much energy." Then I went back into my cave for the last time, packed up my meager possessions, put on my backpack, and said good-bye to my bees and the little brown bird. I was on a high, and I was unconcerned about the several-mile walk back to the other cave. It was a hot desert day, but I was carrying a little water with me. What could go wrong?

Well, when you get too cocky, life has a way of express mailing you a lesson in humility. I found my way out of the canyon to a dirt road, and then I made a wrong turn. I didn't know the territory, and

I headed for a nearby small mountain where I thought the shaman would be. As I searched for the trail I knew led to the cave, I found no trail at all. Just cactus and rough terrain. I climbed rock ledges, watching out for rattlesnakes. The sun beat down on my neck, and I was grateful for my hat. I drank half my water. When I got to the top of the mountain, there was no cave: I had climbed the wrong mountain.

There was almost no phone signal out there, and my battery was nearly dead. Fortunately, I'd had enough experience as a hiker that I didn't panic. I called the shaman, tried to explain where I was, but "on a mountain in the desert, and I can see cactus" isn't very descriptive. Still, I marveled at the strange energy coursing through my body, shattering my limited view of what my body could handle. I knew I could walk all day if I needed to. I climbed back down the mountain, enjoying the red cliffs, looking for a trail. There was no shade to give me a break from the intense desert sun, but I felt so good. I didn't even think about food once.

I was still Dave Asprey, standing alone on top of a craggy hilltop in Arizona, but I was not the same Dave Asprey who had arrived at Delilah's ranch four days earlier, dubious and full of anxieties. The old me had believed, at an instinctual level, that four days without food would create weakness and unbearable hunger. That four days without human contact would stir up crushing sadness and loneliness. I had gone through some rough periods, true, but I had more energy now than before I had started the vision quest. I felt almost giddy. In hindsight, I know exactly what was going on: I had gone into ketosis, so I was burning fat and delivering concentrated energy to my brain. My body was also in a superclean state by then. There were no toxins in my body left over from eating inflammatory fats or proteins or sugar, so there were no digestion by-products clogging my brain.

Those are now well-documented effects of fasting, and it's obvious that they were connected to the things I was feeling. But without a doubt there was a third thing going on: I had just experienced my first true spiritual fast. I still carried the scars of the old me, including the dozens of stretch marks left from the years when I had been seriously overweight, but I didn't care about them as much anymore, and I appreciated the muscle that was emerging beneath them. The past held less of a pull on me than the future. Everyone should have a chance to experience this state, in which you feel absolutely free to live life on your own terms.

There was no cell signal at the top of the next hill or the second. I ended up walking something like ten miles in desert heat with a backpack and a mostly empty bottle of water, by myself after four days of fasting, and I was completely fine. It was crazy, and it was the best hike of my life. I felt so damn good.

I kept going, letting the universe take me wherever it wanted me to go, knowing that I was more than strong enough to handle whatever the universe brought me. And the universe delivered. I found Delilah right as my phone ran out of charge.

BE THE BEST MIRROR TO THE WORLD

As a kid I was an avid reader, and one of my favorite books was *Homer Price*,[1] a collection of stories by the brilliant writer Robert McCloskey. In one of the stories, a traveling salesman named Professor Atmos P. H. Ear comes to town hawking an astonishing product called "Ever-So-Much-More-So" powder. You can sprinkle it on anything, and it makes it more of what it is. So you spread it on a squeaky wheel, it gets more squeaky. If you spread it on a beautiful tree, it gets more beautiful. It's an empty can, of course, but people want to believe. The joke of the story is that Professor Atmos P. H. Ear is both a con artist and a sage. The beauty of the story is that people love his idea so much that they actually begin to see the ever-so-much-more-so effect.

Intermittent fasting acts like the Ever-So-Much-More-So powder. It enables you to be more of who you are and who you want to be. Fasting doesn't guarantee that you'll make the right choices. If you're already kind of a jerk, you'll have more energy to be a jerk. You'll probably end up yelling at people even more than you did before. But if you're earnestly working on making something good happen in your life, your community, or anywhere else in the world, you will do more of that, too. Fasting removes a lot of the obstacles in your way.

One of the things in your way is all the energy you use to think about food. That misplaced fixation removes your peak abilities. If you're always eating and digesting, some portion of you is always doing that thinking—or digesting—instead of doing something else. The pauses when your metabolism gets a rest are the times when your peak experiences can happen.

Step one in a meaningful fast is getting started. You have to push past all the obstacles that block people from even experimenting with fasting: "I might starve, it sounds like torture, it's inconvenient, it's weird, I might fail." You are deeply programmed to avoid death and starvation, and fasting (or even thinking about fasting) will set off those fears. You need to put your modern, rational brain in charge of your ancient, instinctual lizard brain. Step two is using the fast to help you push past all the other obstacles in your life—the ones that prevent you from daring to travel or create or start a family or just be a better version of yourself.

I want you to examine your preconceptions about food and fasting and investigate where they come from. Why do you think they are true? What if a lot of them aren't? Which ones can you actually prove? Many people resist fasting for even one day because of all the emotions it stirs up. They're terrified because they don't know what will happen. Well, here's what's going to happen: You are going to face the hunger. You are also going to face the fact that you may even choose to sit in a room full of people having a social experience called *dinner*, and that your plate is going to be empty. What emotional strings will the voice in your head play then? Is it going to say that you're lonely, you're not part of the group? Yes, it's very likely to say those things. It's lying.

Years after my vision quest at First Woman cave, I was invited to dinner at Kensington Palace in London. I was part of a group of senior executives who were meeting with some European elites. All very proper. As the tuxedo-clad waiters began bringing around waves of fancy food—the kind you'd expect to see served at a palace—I looked around to see what other people were doing. I had politely declined most of the food offered. I like to intermittent fast during business trips and would regularly fast for twenty-four hours around long flights to help prevent jet lag. Still, it seemed socially unacceptable to refuse everything offered to me at Kensington Palace, so I chose a few dinner items to be polite.

Amid all of the clinking of forks on plates, I was intrigued to see that the person seated next to me—Phil Libin, the CEO of Evernote— had nothing on his plate. I asked him what was going on. "I'm fasting," he answered. He told me he was on day three of a five-day fast. He had just lost 80 pounds using fasts of up to eight days and ketosis. Back then, I couldn't comprehend the idea of fasting at a lavish event like this, and I told him so. His response was that he traveled so much that the only way he could build fasting into his life was to decide that he simply was not going to eat, no matter where he was in the world. That totally resonated with me.

So we sat there with his empty plate and my half-empty plate, and we made conversation. You should have seen the reactions of the other people at the table. They were looking at him as though he was going to die. There was definitely judgment coming from people who had absolutely no reason to judge him. I overheard some people spec- ulating that he had an eating disorder, even though he went through the meal perfectly happy and social.

I had a totally different take on what I was witnessing: "Good for you, man. You're doing what you want to do." He had the courage to fuel his own body in a way that works for him, and there are few things as precious as losing 80 or 100 pounds. You may have seen a similar reaction to Jack Dorsey, the CEO of Twitter and Square. We first communicated years ago about his intermittent fasting and coffee habits. Clearly, fasting has worked very well for him. Few humans can be CEO of two public companies at the same time. He says his diet is crucial for being able to pull that off. When he spoke openly about his use of one meal a day (OMAD) fasting, some media outlets tried to frame it as an eating disorder, just as people did with Phil Libin at the dinner party in Kensington Palace. When your diet owns you, it's an eating disorder. When you own your diet, it's part of how you manage your life. There is no way I could run a large podcast, write a book like this every year or two, and also be CEO of two companies if I did not practice fasting. It simply isn't optional if I'm going to have the energy left at the end of the day to also be a good husband, father, and friend.

It's almost as if the hungry voice in other people's heads gets triggered when you decide not to eat. That may, in fact, be exactly what's happening. Mirror neurons may make other people feel hunger when they see that you aren't eating. That response once served an important adaptive function by making sure that hunters shared their kill with the rest of the group and by encouraging the whole clan to eat together and maintain their social bond. Today, however, it's a cruel fact of nature that when *you* choose not to eat for your health, others often interpret your abstaining as *their* pain.

You might also be activating a social type of mirroring: when you make the choice not to eat, it can trigger other people's insecurities about their own eating habits (especially since we live in a culture in which so much shame is attached to food and body weight). Insecure people tend to operate without a lot of generosity; they may subconsciously or even overtly attempt to sabotage your efforts. You can do better, however. Once you understand where these impulses come from, you can handle any detractors with less judgment and more empathy.

I experienced these mirroring effects firsthand on a recent flight from Seattle to Dubai as I was writing this book. It's quite a long flight, about eighteen hours in the air, and I was looking forward to the uninterrupted writing time. Once again, I was fasting on the flight to help stave off jet lag. As I sat down in first class (it's expensive, but it also helps with jet lag), a flight attendant came around to offer me a menu. I smiled and told her that I didn't need a menu because I wasn't going to eat on the flight but that I'd love lots of sparkling water. Her eyes got big, and she insisted on handing me the menu, telling me I would need it when I changed my mind later. I explained that I really didn't want the menu. She looked at me skeptically, as if she thought I might die if I didn't eat for eighteen hours.

Those mirror neurons had her so worried that she recruited another flight attendant to try to get me to take a menu. Fortunately, the new flight attendant, Jacquie, was practicing intermittent fasting and used the Bulletproof Diet to help her handle the grueling demands of her job. She got me. Jacquie was happy to keep the menu and even supported my fast by brewing some coffee (with Bulletproof beans!) for me with a little butter in it.

One lesson I take away from such experiences is that fasting is so scary to the deep parts of our brains that we feel other people's hunger and act to prevent it, often by sabotaging our own fasts or others'. But I also believe that empathy must work both ways. By letting the fast make you a better person and by radiating empathy into the world, you can lift up the people around you.

SET YOURSELF UP FOR SUCCESS

In the first century CE, the Greek Stoic philosopher Epictetus wrote, "We must undergo a hard winter training and not rush into things for which we haven't prepared."[2] I appreciate Stoic philosophy because it addresses the challenges we choose to undertake, and the ways we prepare to face them, in ways that remain fully relevant to the modern world.

There is something to be said for a philosophy centered around enduring unavoidable hardship without complaint while constantly seeking a place of greater virtue. Whether you want to know about fasting or about how to become a highly resilient human, going back to ancient writings can help you get to the source of great truths. I read Ryan Holiday and Stephen Hanselman's *The Daily Stoic: 366 Meditations on Wisdom, Perseverance, and the Art of Living*[3] with my ten-year-old son in the sauna every morning while writing this book. Another quote comes to mind. "You have power over your mind—not outside events," wrote the Roman Stoic Marcus Aurelius in *Meditations*, his seminal work. "Realize this, and you will find strength."

Fasting teaches you how to summon up that power over your mind, whether it's fasting from cigarettes, fasting from alcohol, fasting from porn (which consumes an inordinate amount of some people's energy), or fasting from anything else you purposefully choose to go without. You're going into battle against the inner wiring of your body when you decide to fast, so you must undergo a hard winter training. You should go in with your eyes wide open to the obstacles you will face.

If you say, "Oh, this sounds great, I'm so inspired by this book that I'm going on a five-day, water-only fast," while training for a marathon and starting a new company, I can tell you exactly what is going to happen next: You're going to fail. You might even end up in the hospital.

Set yourself up for success. Getting your body metabolically flexible before you try the big stuff is the best strategy. Start with fasting by using the hacks I've outlined in this book: MCT oil, Bulletproof Coffee, sleep training, exercise training, and controlled breathing, combined in ways that make sense given your physical state and your life situation. Don't push yourself over the edge, but don't overlook any possible advantages, either. Don't rush into things for which you haven't prepared. This is good life advice for any situation but especially for fasting.

I hope you'll indulge my sharing one more quote from Epictetus 2.10.1, as told by Ryan Holiday: "Consider who you are. Above all, a human being, carrying no greater power than your own reasoned choice, which oversees all other things, and is free."[4] Epictetus, who was born a slave, was not given his freedom until the age of eighteen. Words about freedom and reasoned choice have extra power coming from a man who once had neither freedom nor choice.

Going without, which is at the core of fasting, puts you in charge of your own freedom. It's a big task, but if you live the rest of your life controlled by, pushed by, and ultimately allowing cravings and desires to be your puppet masters, you'll never reach your full potential. I doubt that's all you want from life. If you want to rise up and show yourself that you can say no for a little while, well within the safety tolerances of your body, you'll show your body who's boss. And the one who is the boss is you.

Many people talk about diet and fasting as if they are superficial pursuits, inward-looking obsessions in which people care only about being thin and looking healthy while not paying attention to the rest of the world. That is the exact opposite of the truth. If you want to bring something good into the world, you need the energy and focus to be able to turn it from idea into action. Fasting helps you get that energy and focus. It gives you the "Ever-So-Much-More-So" powder that lets you engage with the world as it is and make it into more of the world as it *should be*.

Hold on; we aren't done with Stoic philosophy just yet. Here's what Seneca the Younger, often considered the greatest of the Stoic philosophers, wrote nearly two thousand years ago in his *Moral Letters to Lucilius*, as paraphrased by Ryan Holiday. He argued that "there is no reason to live and no limit to our miseries if we let our fears predominate."[5] If that idea sounds vaguely familiar, there's a reason: Franklin Delano Roosevelt loosely rephrased it as "We have nothing to fear but fear itself." I got a humbling lesson about that when I freaked out over an imaginary mountain lion during my vision quest in the cave.

You now know the biology of fasting, and you know that it's not going to kill you. In fact, if you're doing it right, it won't even be unpleasant. All the same, you probably don't fully accept that truth yet because you haven't experienced it. As long as fear remains in control, it defines your reality. Of the four F's—fear, food, f*cking, and friends—fear is the most powerful. Even things that your rational brain knows are ridiculously, obviously not life-threatening activate the primal biological responses that are designed to prevent you from being killed. That's why fear gets into the way of everything you strive to achieve as a human being, even something as silly as singing karaoke in a bar.

Your body will use that survival instinct to make sure you stuff your face with sugar and whatever else is nearby, because it wants to make sure you don't go without the second F, which is food. It doesn't care whether the food is good for you or not. All it cares about is that you don't run out of energy. So it connects the first and second F's with the fourth one—friends—making the act of eating a warm communal occurrence.

As for the third F, well, there's a reason it often happens after a dinner date. The sensual pleasures and essential acts of survival and reproduction are all scrambled together in our brains. But fear is so intense that it will even overwhelm the third F. Have you ever seen someone really attractive and really wanted to ask him or her out but then didn't have the guts to walk over and introduce yourself? That's fear. It's telling you you're not that person's equal in looks, sexuality, humor, wealth—you name it.

Are you going to endure that fear? Are you going to let it run you, as if you were still standing defenseless on the savanna in front of a hungry tiger? If so, as Seneca says, there will be no limit to your miseries. Find the thing that is the most important to you, the thing that is the most scary, the thing you honestly believe you could never go without for any length of time. Then fast from *that*. Go without, even if for just one day. Just long enough to make you uncomfortable. Then look in the mirror and see if you like the person who's there.

I promise you that you'll like that person better than you did before. That is the magic of fasting.

YOUR NEXT FAST (AND THE ONE AFTER THAT)

Throughout this book, I've shared my experience of the vision quest in the cave as an inspirational tale, but also as a cautionary one. When you fast from something, especially at the beginning, the volume and frequency of the noises in your head will increase. They will go from hidden whispers—soft, gentle tones you wouldn't notice unless you were deep in meditation—to distinct, audible complaints. Then to shouts. Then to screams. Then, finally, you'll hear raw panic fully exposed.

When the voices are at their most extreme and dramatic, that's also when you can finally hear just how false they ring. The secret of fasting, which is also the secret of owning your own biology and your own life, is developing ways to separate truth from fiction. Your body lies to you, but it's nothing personal. Its lies have evolved over millions of years as useful instincts to keep you alive. You wouldn't be here today without them. Your body also tells you the truth sometimes. Once you understand that these messages are ancient adaptations to help you survive conditions you no longer face, you can begin to separate needs from wants and truths from lies.

Anyone who knows me well, or who reads my books and blogs regularly, knows that I have a distaste for certain words I call "weasel words." These are important-sounding words that have loose, malleable definitions. People use such language when they're not quite sure what they want to say—or when they don't want to take responsibility for a clear opinion. We've all probably relied on them at times to muddle through business meetings or to wriggle out of uncomfortable situations; I sure have. But they can easily lead to dishonesty, confusion, and inaction.

Need, to me, is a weasel word. It's the most overused word in the English language, yet it is almost always untrue. The way to differentiate between a *need* and a *want* is to add the words "or I will die" to the end of the sentence. Then check to see if your "need" statement is still true. Most of the things we casually say that we need ("I need that iPhone! I need that shirt!") aren't needs at all. Saying that we "need" them endows all kinds of unnecessary things with power over us.

So here's a different kind of fasting challenge: fast for just one day from words that make you weak. Language influences how we think and how we feel. If you master the word *need* and you stop using it in misleading and disempowering ways, every other fast you attempt will become magically easier. If you really want to spice things up, promise your spouse, your friends, your coworkers, or your kids that you'll donate $5 to a charity each time you use the words *need* and *can't*, another ubiquitous weasel word. At the end of the day, you will probably be wondering how exactly you're going to foot the bill you just created for yourself.

Or you could try another very useful type of linguistic fast: tell yourself that you will use only truthful language today. It's really challenging, harder even than you probably imagine. As part of your fast from falsehood, fast from the word *can't*. This means that the next time someone asks you, "Hey, can you pick me up at the airport?" and you're not in the mood, you want to find a way to tell them you would love to but you just ___. Oops. Or when someone asks you to meet for lunch and you tell them, with apologies, that you'd love to but just ___.

When you say you can't do those things, you're a liar. The honest truth—the reality—is that of course you could. You could cancel everything else and go to that lunch. You could take an hour off work and drive to the airport. So why do you say you can't when you can and just choose not to? Maybe you're trying to protect people's feelings. Maybe. Or more likely, it makes you uncomfortable to stand up for yourself and say directly what you want and don't want to do. Try it for a day and notice how different you feel. Hold on: *do* it for a day and notice how different you feel. (*Try* is another weasel word, a way to pretend you are going to do something that you probably never will.) If you're worried about offending people, tell your friends that you're going on a lying fast. For one day, you will tell no lies, no matter how small. They might think you're crazy, but it will be easier if you're truthful about it. It's as liberating to learn to go a day without lying as it is to go a day without food.

Fasting from food is an entry point into an enormous, powerful world of honesty and control. As soon as you stop hiding in one part of your life, all kinds of other possibilities begin to open up. That's why I've written this book. It's not about helping you fit into your bathing suit or reducing your risk of atherosclerosis—though they certainly are nice bonuses. I want to invite you to open up the possibility of radical self-improvement.

Start by giving up the word *can't*. Walk away from saying "need" unless you're describing something that you genuinely, desperately do need and will perish without. These seemingly tiny challenges are incredibly difficult. But if you can remove those two words from your vocabulary for a day, you can also go a day without food. You can fast from hate. You can put more kindness and generosity into the world. You can be the true master of *you*.

Language may be the most powerful biohack of all. If you want to ease into your first fast with a cup of Bulletproof Coffee, that's fine. I love it, I use it, and I will happily sell it to you. But whatever kind of fast you are planning, you will have a much greater chance of success if you work on the voices in your head first, because it will make the whole process so much easier. You will become aware of the difference between a want and a need, between a fear and a genuine danger. When you actually fast and get far into it—to the stage at which things would be going horribly wrong for if your fears were correct—that's when the voices in your head will tend to go really, really quiet. Then you will know the blissful silence that I discovered for the first time at the end of my vision quest.

In the end, fasting not only brings you physical improvements, mental clarity, emotional openness, and spiritual insight, it also brings you stillness. It brings you peace. Ultimately, that is my wish for you: *May your next fast, and the fast after that, bring you peace.*

Don't be afraid to go without. It will change your life.

ACKNOWLEDGMENTS

Every time I tell my family I want to write another book, it is with mixed feelings. My wife, Lana, and my kids, Anna and Alan, know that when there is a book in my brain ready to come out, it's for a good cause, and they know that the longer I wait when a book is ready, the more stressful it gets. I am grateful they were supportive and understanding of all the late nights and deadlines that come on top of my normal life hosting *Bulletproof Radio* and running my other companies. Likewise, the people who run the companies in my portfolio know that when I go into writing mode, I am asking more of them because my brain will be somewhere else for a little while. First, I'd like to thank my family for making time and space for me to do this, on top of my other responsibilities, and I'd like to thank my team for their support while I do this.

There's a romantic view of the lone author locked in a room somewhere writing books, but that's not really how it works. Writing a book that is more than worth the time it takes to write and the time it takes to read is a team sport. The reason this book is the way it is now is my amazing editor, Julie Will at Harper Wave; my writing partner for this book, Corey Powell; and Celeste Fine, my agent. All of them have had so many amazing suggestions to make the book the finest possible. Thanks to Bev Hampson, who managed my packed calendar and made sure I hit my deadlines and still had time to walk the talk and take care of myself while also being an active husband, father, CEO, author, and podcaster.

Special thanks to my teams at TrueDark, 40 Years of Zen, Home-biotic and The Dave Asprey Box, Upgrade Labs, and my coaching institute, The Human Potential Institute.

I first wrote about intermittent fasting in 2010, and it was a part of my life for several years before that. Since then, so much new knowledge has come out and I am grateful to have had the opportunity to talk to many of the world's top experts on fasting, who have helped me figure out the details, taught me along the way, and shared this knowledge with the world, including Jason Fung, Jimmy Moore, Naomi Whittel, Mark Mattson, Brad Pilon, Mark Sisson, Wim Hof, Dr. Joseph Mercola, Dr. Amy Shah, Dr. Sylvia Tara, Siim Land, Dr. Rudy Tanzi, Dr. Molly Maloof, Dr. David Sinclair, Dr. David Perl-mutter, Tina Anderson, James Clement, Chalene Johnson, Naveen Jain, Michael Platt, J. J. Virgin, Satchin Panda, Matt Gallant, and Wade Lightheart.

Special thanks to a few friends who share extra business support and wisdom: Joe Polish's Genius Network, J. J. Virgin's Mindshare Group, Michael Fishman's Consumer Health Summit, and Dan Sullivan's Strategic Coach.

Assuming you are reading this, I would like to acknowledge you, for investing your time and attention in this book. I sincerely hope it was more than worth the time you put into it.

Happy Fasting!

NOTES

PROLOGUE: FASTING TO FIND YOUR BEST SELF

1. Mark S. George and Jeffrey P. Lorberbaum, "Sexual Function," in *Encyclopedia of the Human Brain*, ed. V. S. Ramachandran (New York: Academic Press, 2002), vol. 1, 355–65.

I: FASTING IS ONLY IN YOUR HEAD

1. Berthold Laufer, "Origin of the Word Shaman," *American Anthropologist* New Series 19, no. 3 (July–September 1917): 361–37, https://www.jstor.org/stable/660223?seq=1#metadata_info_tab_contents.

2. Hun-young Park et al., "The Effects of Altitude/Hypoxic Training on Oxygen Delivery Capacity of the Blood and Aerobic Exercise Capacity in Elite Athletes—a Meta-analysis," *Journal of Exercise Nutrition and Biochemistry* 20, no. 1 (March 2016): 15–22, https://www.ncbi.nlm.nih.gov/pmc/articles/PMC4899894.

3. Cameron Sepah, "The Definitive Guide to Dopamine Fasting 2.0: The Hot Silicon Valley Trend," The Startup, October 28, 2019, https://medium.com/swlh/dopamine-fasting-2-0-the-hot-silicon-valley-trend-7c4dc3ba2213.

4. Alison Moodie, "The Complete Intermittent Fasting Guide for Beginners," Bulletproof, December 5, 2019, https://www.bulletproof.com/diet/intermittent-fasting/intermittent-fasting-guide.

5. Adrienne R. Barnosky et al., "Intermittent Fasting vs Daily Calorie Restriction for Type 2 Diabetes Prevention: A Review of Human Findings," *Translational Research* 164, no. 4 (October 2014): 302–11, https://www.sciencedirect.com/science/article/pii/S193152441400200X.

6. Danielle Glick, Sandra Barth, and Kay F. Macleod, "Autophagy: Cellular and Molecular Mechanisms," *Journal of Pathology* 221, no. 2 (May 2010): 3–12, https://www.ncbi.nlm.nih.gov/pmc/articles/PMC2990190.

7. Mehrdad Alirezaei et al., "Short-Term Fasting Induces Profound Neuronal Autophagy," *Autophagy* 6, no. 6 (August 2010): 702–10, https://pubmed.ncbi.nlm.nih.gov/20534972.

8. Takayuki Teruya et al., "Diverse metabolic reactions activated during 58-hr fasting are revealed by non-targeted metabolomic analysis of human blood," *Scientific Reports* 9, no. 854 (2019), https://www.nature.com/articles/s41598-018-36674-9.

9. Maria M. Mihaylova et al., "Fasting Activates Fatty Acid Oxidation to Enhance Intestinal Stem Cell Function During Homeostasis and Aging," *Cell Stem Cell* 22, no. 5 (May 2018): 769–78, https://www.cell.com/cell-stem-cell/pdfExtended/S1934-5909(18)30163-2.

10. Dave Asprey, *The Bulletproof Diet: Lose Up to a Pound a Day, Reclaim Energy and Focus, Upgrade Your Life* (New York: Rodale Books, 2014).

11. Amandine Chaix and Satchidananda Panda, "Ketone Bodies Signal Opportunistic Food-Seeking Activity," *Trends in Endocrinology & Metabolism* 27, no. 6 (March 2016): 350–52, https://www.ncbi.nlm.nih.gov/pmc/articles/PMC4903165.

12. Camille Vandenberghe et al., "Caffeine Intake Increases Plasma Ketones: An Acute Metabolic Study in Humans," *Canadian Journal of Physiology and Pharmacology* 95, no. 4 (2017): 455–58, https://www.nrcresearchpress.com/doi/10.1139/cjpp-2016-0338#.X0cYZ-d7mUk.

13. C. G. Proud, "Amino Acids and mTOR Signalling in Anabolic Function," *Biochemical Society Transactions* 35, no. 5 (November 2007): 1187–90, https://portlandpress.com/biochemsoctrans/article-abstract/35/5/1187/85681/Amino-acids-and-mTOR-signalling-in-anabolic?redirectedFrom=fulltext.

14. V. V. Frolkis et al., "Enterosorption in Prolonging Old Animal Lifespan," *Experimental Gerontology* 19, no. 4 (February 1984): 217–25, https://www.researchgate.net/publication/223057524_Enterosorption_in_prolonging_old_animal_lifespan.

15. Ron Sender, Shai Fuchs, and Ron Milo, "Revised Estimates for the Number of Human and Bacteria Cells in the Body," *PLOS Biology* 14, no. 8 (August 2016): e1002533, https://www.ncbi.nlm.nih.gov/pmc/articles/PMC4991899.

16. Amanda Gardner, "Soluble and Insoluble Fiber: What's the Difference?," WebMD, July 23, 2015, https://www.webmd.com/diet/features/insoluble -soluble-fiber.

17. "Alcohol's Effects on the Body," National Institute on Alcohol Abuse and Alcoholism, https://www.niaaa.nih.gov/alcohols-effects-health/alcohols-effects -body.

18. Ian McLaughlin, John A. Dani, and Mariella De Biasi, "Nicotine With-drawal," in *Current Topics in Behavioral Neurosciences*, vol. 24, *The Neuro-biology and Genetics of Nicotine and Tobacco*, ed. David J. K. Balfour and Marcus R. Munafò (New York: Springer, 2015), 99–123, https://link .springer.com/chapter/10.1007%2F978-3-319-13482-6_4.

2: ENLISTING YOUR MOLECULAR MACHINES

1. "Celsus, *De Medicina*," http://penelope.uchicago.edu/Thayer/E/Roman /Texts/Celsus/home.html.

2. "Chemicals in Meat Cooked at High Temperatures and Cancer Risk," National Cancer Institute, July 11, 2017, https://www.cancer.gov/about -cancer/causes-prevention/risk/diet/cooked-meats-fact-sheet.

3. Dave Asprey, "The Complete Bulletproof Diet Roadmap," https://blog .daveasprey.com/the-complete-illustrated-one-page-bulletproof-diet.

4. Yang Luo and Song Guo Zheng, "Hall of Fame Among Pro-inflammatory Cytokines: Interleukin-6 Gene and Its Transcriptional Regulation Mecha-nisms," *Frontiers in Immunology* 7 (2016): 604, https://www.frontiersin.org /articles/10.3389/fimmu.2016.00604/full.

5. "Cardiovascular Diseases (CVDs)," World Health Organization, May 17, 2017, https://www.who.int/news-room/fact-sheets/detail/cardiovascular-diseases -(cvds).

6. Kimberley J. Smith et al., "The Association Between Loneliness, Social Isolation and Inflammation: A Systematic Review and Meta-analysis," *Neuroscience & Biobehavioral Reviews* 112 (May 2020): 519–41, https://www .sciencedirect.com/science/article/abs/pii/S0149763419308292?via%3Dihub.

7. "New England Centenarian Study," BU School of Medicine, http://www .bumc.bu.edu/centenarian.

8. Mikhail V. Blagosklonny, "Hormesis Does Not Make Sense Except in the Light of TOR-Driven Aging," *Aging* 3, no. 11 (November 2011): 1051–62, https://www.ncbi.nlm.nih.gov/pmc/articles/PMC3249451.

9. Zhenyu Zhong et al., "New mitochondrial DNA synthesis enables NLRP3 inflammasome activation," *Nature* 560 (July 2018): 198–203, https://www.ncbi.nlm.nih.gov/pmc/articles/PMC6329306.

3: MANY STAGES AND MANY STYLES OF FASTING

1. Select Committee on Nutrition and Human Needs, United States Senate, *Dietary Goals for the United States*, 2nd ed. (Washington, DC: U.S. Government Printing Office, 1977), https://naldc.nal.usda.gov/download/1759572/PDF.

2. Leah M. Kalm and Richard D. Semba, "They Starved So That Others Be Better Fed: Remembering Ancel Keys and the Minnesota Experiment," *The Journal of Nutrition* 135, no. 6 (June 2005): 1347–52, https://academic.oup.com/jn/article/135/6/1347/4663828.

3. Kim S. Stote et al., "A Controlled Trial of Reduced Meal Frequency Without Caloric Restriction in Healthy, Normal-Weight, Middle-Aged Adults," *American Journal of Clinical Nutrition* 85, no. 4 (April 2007): 981–88, https://www.ncbi.nlm.nih.gov/pmc/articles/PMC2645638.

4. Alan Goldhamer et al., "Medically Supervised Water-Only Fasting in the Treatment of Hypertension," *Journal of Manipulative and Physiological Therapeutics* 24, no. 5 (June 2001): 335–39, https://www.jmptonline.org/article/S0161-4754(01)85575-5/fulltext.

5. Alessio Nencioni et al., "Fasting and Cancer: Molecular Mechanisms and Clinical Application," *Nature Reviews Cancer* 18 (2018): 707–19, https://www.nature.com/articles/s41568-018-0061-0.

4: FAST FOR LONG LIFE

1. Kathleen Holder, "Moroccan Fossils Show Human Ancestors' Diet of Game," UC Davis, June 7, 2017, https://www.ucdavis.edu/news/moroccan-fossils-show-human-ancestors-diet-game.

2. Alexandra Rosati, "Food for Thought: Was Cooking a Pivotal Step in Human Evolution?," *Scientific American*, February 26, 2018, https://www.scientificamerican.com/article/food-for-thought-was-cooking-a-pivotal-step-in-human-evolution.

3. Abigail Carroll, *Three Squares: The Invention of the American Meal* (New York: Basic Books, 2013).

4. Mark P. Mattson, "Challenging Oneself Intermittently to Improve Health," *Dose-Response* 12, no. 4 (December 2014): 600–18, https://www.ncbi.nlm.nih.gov/pmc/articles/PMC4267452/pdf/drp-12-600.pdf.

5. "Diabetes," World Health Organization, June 8, 2020, https://www.who.int/news-room/fact-sheets/detail/diabetes.

6. Edward Hooker Dewey, *The True Science of Living* (Norwich, CT: The Henry Bill Publishing Company, 1895), https://openlibrary.org/works/OL10331648W/The_true_science_of_living, 171.

7. Claude Bélanger, "Fasting by Canadian Indians," The Quebec History Encyclopedia: 2004, http://faculty.marianopolis.edu/c.belanger/quebechistory/encyclopedia/IndianFasting.htm.

8. D. W. Reiff and K. K. L. Reiff, "Time Spent Thinking About Food," *Healthy Weight Journal* (1998): 84.

9. Bec Crew, "Your Appendix Might Serve an Important Biological Function After All," ScienceAlert, January 10, 2017, https://www.sciencealert.com/your-appendix-might-serve-an-important-biological-function-after-all-2.

10. Anne Trafton, "A New Player in Appetite Control. Brain Cells That Provide Structural Support Also Influence Feeding Behavior, Study Shows," MIT News, October 18, 2016, http://news.mit.edu/2016/brain-cells-structural-support-influence-appetite-1018.

11. Sang-Ha Baik et al., "Intermittent Fasting Increases Adult Hippocampal Neurogenesis," *Brain and Behavior* 10, no. 1 (January 2020): e01444, https://onlinelibrary.wiley.com/doi/full/10.1002/brb3.1444.

12. Krisztina Marosi and Mark P. Mattson, "BDNF Mediates Adaptive Brain and Body Responses to Energetic Challenges," *Trends in Endocrinology & Metabolism* 25, no. 2 (2014): 89–98, https://www.ncbi.nlm.nih.gov/pmc/articles/PMC3915771.

13. Aiwu Cheng et al., "Mitochondrial SIRT3 Mediates Adaptive Responses of Neurons to Exercise and Metabolic and Excitatory Challenges," *Cell Metabolism* 23, no. 1 (January 2016): 128–42, https://www.cell.com/cell-metabolism/fulltext/S1550-4131(15)00529-X.

14. Jeong Seon Yoon et al., "3,6'-dithiothalidomide improves experimental stroke outcome by suppressing neuroinflammation," *Journal of Neuroscience Research* 91, no. 5 (February 2013), https://onlinelibrary.wiley.com/doi/abs/10.1002/jnr.23190.

15. Bae Kun Shin et al., "Intermittent Fasting Protects Against the Deterioration of Cognitive Function, Energy Metabolism and Dyslipidemia in Alzheimer's Disease–Induced Estrogen Deficient Rats," *Experimental Biology and Medicine* 243, no. 4 (February 2018): 334–43, https://www.ncbi.nlm.nih.gov/pmc/articles/PMC6022926.

16. Bob Grant, "Running on Empty," *The Scientist*, May 31, 2017, https://www.the-scientist.com/features/running-on-empty-31436.

5: FAST FOR BETTER SLEEP; SLEEP FOR A BETTER FAST

1. Alex C. Keene and Erik R. Duboue, "The Origins and Evolution of Sleep," *Journal of Experimental Biology* 221 (2018): jeb159533, https://jeb.biologists.org/content/221/11/jeb159533.

2. Jeremy Rehm, "World's First Animal Was a Pancake-Shaped Prehistoric Ocean Dweller," *Nature*, September 20, 2018, https://www.nature.com/articles/d41586-018-06767-6.

3. Carol A. Everson, Bernard M. Bergmann, and Allan Rechtschaffen, "Sleep Deprivation in the Rat: III. Total Sleep Deprivation," *Sleep* 12, no. 1 (February 1989): 13–21, https://pubmed.ncbi.nlm.nih.gov/2928622.

4. Natalie L. Hauglund, Chiara Pavan, and Maiken Nedergaard, "Cleaning the Sleeping Brain—the Potential Restorative Function of the Glymphatic System," *Current Opinion in Physiology* 15 (June 2020): 1–6, https://www.sciencedirect.com/science/article/pii/S2468867319301609.

5. "Short Sleep Duration Among US Adults," Centers for Disease Control and Prevention, https://www.cdc.gov/sleep/data_statistics.html.

6. Ruth E. Patterson and Dorothy D. Sears, "Metabolic Effects of Intermittent Fasting," *Annual Review of Nutrition* 37 (August 2017): 371–93, https://www.annualreviews.org/doi/abs/10.1146/annurev-nutr-071816-064634.

7. "The Nobel Prize in Physiology or Medicine 2017," press release, The Nobel Foundation, October 2, 2017, https://www.nobelprize.org/prizes/medicine/2017/press-release.

8. Maria Comas et al., "A Circadian Based Inflammatory Response—Implications for Respiratory Disease and Treatment," *Sleep Science and Practice* 1, no. 18 (2017), https://sleep.biomedcentral.com/articles/10.1186/s41606-017-0019-2.

9. Paul Gringras et al., "Bigger, Brighter, Bluer-Better? Current light-emitting devices—adverse sleep properties and preventative strategies," *Frontiers in*

Public Health (October 2015), https://www.frontiersin.org/articles/10.3389/fpubh.2015.00233/full.

10. Naresh M. Punjabi, "The Epidemiology of Adult Obstructive Sleep Apnea," *Proceedings of the American Thoracic Society* 5, no. 2 (February 15, 2008): 136–43, https://www.ncbi.nlm.nih.gov/pmc/articles/PMC2645248.

11. "Losing Tongue Fat Improves Sleep Apnea," Penn Medicine News, January 10, 2020, https://www.pennmedicine.org/news/news-releases/2020/january/losing-tongue-fat-improves-sleep-apnea.

12. Angela Adelizzi, "Obesity and Obstructive Sleep Apnea," Obesity Medicine Association, May 5, 2017, https://obesitymedicine.org/2017/05/05/obesity-and-sleep-apnea.

13. "What Is Restless Legs Syndrome (RLS)?," Johns Hopkins Medicine, https://www.hopkinsmedicine.org/neurology_neurosurgery/centers_clinic/restless-legs-syndrome/what-is-rls.

14. Song Lin et al., "The Association Between Obesity and Restless Legs Syndrome: A Systemic Review and Meta-analysis of Observational Studies," *Journal of Affective Disorders* 235 (August 2018): 384–91, https://pubmed.ncbi.nlm.nih.gov/29674254.

15. M. T. Streppel et al., "Long-Term Wine Consumption Is Related to Cardiovascular Mortality and Life Expectancy Independently of Moderate Alcohol Intake: The Zutphen Study," *Journal of Epidemiology & Community Health* 63, no. 7 (2009): 534–40, https://jech.bmj.com/content/jech/63/7/534.full.pdf.

16. Corby K. Martin et al., "Effect of Calorie Restriction on Mood, Quality of Life, Sleep, and Sexual Function in Healthy Nonobese Adults: The CALERIE 2 Randomized Clinical Trial," *JAMA Internal Medicine* 176, no. 6 (June 2016): 743–52, https://jamanetwork.com/journals/jamainternalmedicine/fullarticle/2517920#ioi160017r18.

17. G. Grizard et al., "Effect of Short-Term Starvation on Leydig Cell Function in Adult Rats," *Archives of Andrology* 38, no. 3 (May–June 1997): 207–14, https://pubmed.ncbi.nlm.nih.gov/9140617.

18. K. Abdullah, M. Al-Habori, and E. Al-Eryani, "Ramadan Intermittent Fasting Affects Adipokines and Leptin/Adiponectin Ratio in Type 2 Diabetes Mellitus and Their First-Degree Relatives," *BioMed Research International* 2020 (July 2020), https://www.hindawi.com/journals/bmri/2020/1281792.

6: FAST FOR FITNESS AND STRENGTH

1. Rachana Kamtekar, "Marcus Aurelius," Stanford Encyclopedia of Philosophy, December 22, 2017, https://plato.stanford.edu/entries/marcus-aurelius.

2. Krisztina Marosi et al., "Metabolic and Molecular Framework for the Enhancement of Endurance by Intermittent Food Deprivation," *The FASEB Journal* 32, no. 7 (July 2018): 3844–58, https://www.ncbi.nlm.nih.gov/pmc/articles/PMC5998977.

3. A. B. Gray, R. D. Telford, and M. J. Weidemann, "Endocrine Response to Intense Interval Exercise," *European Journal of Applied Physiology and Occupational Physiology* 66 (April 1993): 366–71, https://link.springer.com/article/10.1007/BF00237784#page-1.

4. Paul H. Falcone et al., "Caloric Expenditure of Aerobic, Resistance, or Combined High-Intensity Interval Training Using a Hydraulic Resistance System in Healthy Men," *Journal of Strength & Conditioning Research* 29, no. 3 (March 2015): 779–85, https://journals.lww.com/nsca-jscr/Fulltext/2015/03000/Caloric_Expenditure_of_Aerobic,_Resistance,_or.28.aspx.

5. A. Mooventhan and L. Nivethitha, "Scientific Evidence–Based Effects of Hydrotherapy on Various Systems of the Body," *North American Journal of Medical Sciences* 6, no. 5 (May 2014): 199–209, https://www.ncbi.nlm.nih.gov/pmc/articles/PMC4049052.

6. Tanjaniina Laukkanen et al., "Association Between Sauna Bathing and Fatal Cardiovascular and All-Cause Mortality Events," *JAMA Internal Medicine* 175, no. 4 (April 2015): 542–48, https://jamanetwork.com/journals/jamainternalmedicine/fullarticle/2130724.

7. Jari A. Laukkanen, Tanjaniina Laukkanen, and Setor K. Kunutsor, "Cardiovascular and Other Health Benefits of Sauna Bathing: A Review of the Evidence," *Mayo Clinic Proceedings* 93, no. 8 (August 2018): 1111–21, https://www.mayoclinicproceedings.org/article/S0025-6196(18)30275-1/fulltext#%20.

7: FAST FOR MENTAL AND SPIRITUAL HEALTH

1. Roderik J. S. Gerritsen and Guido P. H. Band, "Breath of Life: The Respiratory Vagal Stimulation Model of Contemplative Activity," *Frontiers in Human Neuroscience* 12 (2018): 397, https://www.frontiersin.org/articles/10.3389/fnhum.2018.00397/full.

2. "About Holotropic Breathwork," Grof Transpersonal Training, http://www
.holotropic.com/holotropic-breathwork/about-holotropic-breathwork.

3. Hadley Meares, "The Medieval Prophetess Who Used Her Visions to Criticize the Church," Atlas Obscura, July 13, 2016, https://www.atlasobscura
.com/articles/the-medieval-prophetess-who-used-her-visions-to-criticize
-the-church.

8: SUPPLEMENTS TO FINE-TUNE YOUR BODY

1. David J. Chalmers, "Facing Up to the Problem of Consciousness," *Journal
of Consciousness Studies* 2, no. 3 (1995): 200–19, http://consc.net/papers
/facing.html.

2. Alayna DeMartini, "Higher Carbon Dioxide Levels Prompt More Plant
Growth, but Fewer Nutrients," College of Food, Agricultural, and Environmental Sciences, The Ohio State University, April 3, 2018, https://cfaes
.osu.edu/news/articles/higher-carbon-dioxide-levels-prompt-more-plant
-growth-fewer-nutrients.

3. Jeffrey S. Hampl, Christopher A. Taylor, and Carol S. Johnston, "Vitamin C
Deficiency and Depletion in the United States: The Third National Health
and Nutrition Examination Survey, 1988 to 1994," *American Journal of
Public Health* 94, no. 5 (May 2004): 870–75, https://www.ncbi.nlm.nih
.gov/pmc/articles/PMC1448351.

4. Dana E. King et al., "Dietary Magnesium and C-Reactive Protein Levels,"
Journal of the American College of Nutrition 24, no. 3 (June 2005): 166–71,
https://pubmed.ncbi.nlm.nih.gov/15930481.

9: IT'S A LITTLE DIFFERENT FOR WOMEN

1. Pradeep M. K. Nair and Pranav G. Khawale, "Role of Therapeutic Fasting in Women's Health: An Overview," *Journal of Mid-Life Health* 7, no. 2
(April–June 2016): 61–64, https://www.ncbi.nlm.nih.gov/pmc/articles/PMC
4960941.

2. "Intermittent Fasting: Women vs. Men," ISSA, 2018, https://www.issaonline
.com/blog/index.cfm/2018/this-hot-diet-trend-is-not-recommended
-for-women.

3. Sushil Kumar and Gurcharan Kaur, "Intermittent Fasting Dietary Restriction Regimen Negatively Influences Reproduction in Young Rats: A Study

of Hypothalamo-Hypophysial-Gonadal Axis," *PLOS ONE* 8, no. 1 (January 2013): e52416, https://journals.plos.org/plosone/article?id=10.1371/journal.pone.0052416.

4. Ibid.

5. Bronwen Martin et al., "Sex-Dependent Metabolic, Neuroendocrine, and Cognitive Responses to Dietary Energy Restriction and Excess," *Endocrinology* 148, no. 9 (September 2007): 4318–33, https://pubmed.ncbi.nlm.nih.gov/17569758.

6. Erin Duffin, "Resident Population of the United States by Sex and Age as of July 1, 2019," Statista, July 20, 2020, https://www.statista.com/statistics/241488/population-of-the-us-by-sex-and-age.

7. Sareh Zeydabadi Nejad, Fahimeh Ramezani Tehrani, and Azita Zadeh-Vakili, "The Role of Kisspeptin in Female Reproduction," *International Journal of Endocrinology & Metabolism* 15, no. 3 (2017): e44337, https://www.ncbi.nlm.nih.gov/pmc/articles/PMC5702467.

10: FAST *EVERY* WAY: A HOW-TO GUIDE

1. David Kestenbaum, "Atomic Tune-up: How the Body Rejuvenates Itself," *All Things Considered*, NPR, July 14, 2007, https://www.npr.org/templates/story/story.php?storyId=11893583.

2. Martin Berkhan, "My Transformation," Leangains, https://leangains.com/tag/my-transformation.

3. Ruth E. Patterson et al., "Intermittent Fasting and Human Metabolic Health," *Journal of the Academy of Nutrition and Dietetics* 115, no. 8 (August 2015): 1203–12, https://jandonline.org/article/S2212-2672(15)00205-1/abstract.

4. James B. Johnson, Donald R. Laub, and Sujit John, "The Effect on Health of Alternate Day Calorie Restriction: Eating Less and More than Needed on Alternate Days Prolongs Life," *Medical Hypotheses* 67, no. 2 (2006): 209–11, https://www.sciencedirect.com/science/article/abs/pii/S0306987706000892?via%3Dihub.

5. James B. Johnson et al., "Alternate Day Calorie Restriction Improves Clinical Findings and Reduces Markers of Oxidative Stress and Inflammation in Overweight Adults with Moderate Asthma," *Free Radical Biology and Medicine* 42, no. 5 (March 2007): 665–74, https://www.ncbi.nlm.nih.gov/pmc/articles/PMC1859864.

6. Krista A. Varady et al., "Alternate Day Fasting for Weight Loss in Normal Weight and Overweight Subjects: A Randomized Controlled Trial," *Nutrition Journal* 12, no. 1 (November 12, 2013): article 146, https://nutritionj .biomedcentral.com/articles/10.1186/1475-2891-12-146.

7. Mark P. Mattson, Valter D. Longo, and Michelle Harvie, "Impact of Intermittent Fasting on Health and Disease Processes," *Ageing Research Reviews* 39 (October 2017): 46–58, https://pubmed.ncbi.nlm.nih.gov/27810402.

8. Leonie K. Heilbronn et al., "Glucose Tolerance and Skeletal Muscle Gene Expression in Response to Alternate Day Fasting," *Obesity Research* 13, no. 3 (2012): 574–81, https://onlinelibrary.wiley.com/doi/full/10.1038/oby .2005.61.

9. Min Wei et al., "Fasting-Mimicking Diet and Markers/Risk Factors for Aging, Diabetes, Cancer, and Cardiovascular Disease," *Science Translational Medicine* 9, no. 377 (February 15, 2017): eaai8700, https://stm.sciencemag .org/content/9/377/eaai8700.

CONCLUSION: FAST IN PEACE

1. Robert McCloskey, *Homer Price* (New York: Puffin Books, 2005) (reissue).

2. Ryan Holiday and Stephen Hanselman, *The Daily Stoic: 366 Meditations on Wisdom, Perseverance, and the Art of Living* (New York: Portfolio, 2016).

3. Ibid.

4. Ibid.

5. Ibid.

INDEX

ABOUT THE AUTHOR

DAVE ASPREY is the creator of the hugely popular Bulletproof Coffee and founder of the Bulletproof company. A three-time *New York Times* bestselling author, he hosts the top-100 podcast *Bulletproof Radio* and has been featured in *Men's Health*, *Outside* magazine, *Wired*, and *Vogue*, and on Fox News, *Nightline*, *The Dr. Oz Show*, *The Joe Rogan Experience*, CNN, and hundreds more. Called the "father of biohacking," he's spent the last two decades working alongside world-renowned doctors, researchers, scientists, and mystics to unlock new levels of happiness and mental and physical performance. Dave is also an active investor in the wellness space, and is the founder and CEO of Bulletproof Media, Upgrade Labs, TrueDark, and 40 Years of Zen. For more, visit DaveAsprey.com.